Applied Ethics

2

Graphics by: Mauro Ghilardini
Original photos: Spencer Davis

Phronesis Editore – 90138 Palermo
Series APPLIED ETHICS
https://phronesis.it/
phronesis.editore@gmail.com

First Edition

Fulvio Di Blasi

VACCINATION AS AN ACT OF LOVE?

The Epistemology of Ethical Choice in Times of Pandemic

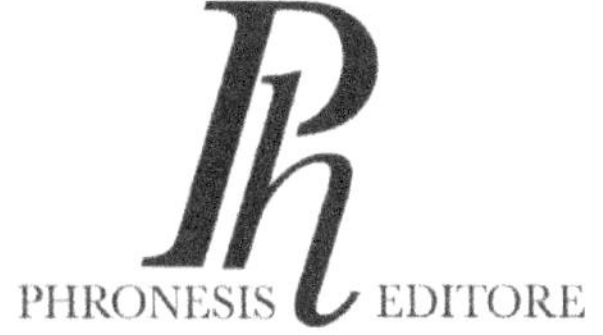

ISBN: 9788897328377

Table of contents

To my wife Francesca
who made so many sacrifices to enable me to write this and
the other volumes of the overall work quickly
and who shared her inspiration and concerns with me

Preface to the English edition

The Italian version of this book was already entirely drafted at the end of 2021, revised at the beginning of 2022, and published in February 2022. So much has occurred since then. Now, for example, after Janine Small's statements to the European Parliament,[1] everyone knows that Covid vaccines do not stop the spread of the virus and cannot create herd immunity. There was no need for the vaccine passport or the vaccine mandate. It's funny that for most people this was a shocking discovery while, as I explain in chapter 5, this was an obvious fact for anyone familiar with the official marketing documents.

Not many know, however, that the most up-to-date scientific data clearly indicate that these "vaccines" are – in many cases and for some age groups – worse than the disease.[2] The adverse ef-

1 For the video of Janine Small's parliamentary question, see Rob Roos' tweet at the link: https://twitter.com/Rob_Roos/status/1579759795225198593?ref_src=twsrc%5Etfw%7Ctwcamp%5Etweetembed%7Ctwterm%5E1579759795225198593%7Ctwgr%5E42a2cf3a876edcceaac251a07c8985b3a159b30f%7Ctwcon%5Es1_&ref_url=https%3A%2F%2Fwww.iltempo.it%2Festeri%2F2022%2F10%2F11%2Fnews%2Fcovid-pfizer-janine-small-parlamento-ue-ammette-non-abbiamo-testato-vaccino-fermare-trasmissione-virus-33420706%2F.

2 See F. Di Blasi (ed.), *Vaccinazioni COVID-19 e Costituzione: evidenza scientifica e analisi etico-giuridica* (Phronesis Editore: Palermo 2022). Especially: M. Bizzarri, "Evidenze scientifiche e criticità dei vaccini," pp. 30-44; L. Teodori, "Miocarditi e Pericarditi post Vaccinazione anti

(continued on the next page)

fects, the increase in total mortality, the weakening of the immune system of the vaccinated, or the fact that the fanaticism of the Covid-19 pandemic has generated wider syndemic problems, are now issues that the real experts know well, even if the mainstream media continue to silence them.

In Italy, at around the same time I was publishing this book, some judges were starting to take courage and refer the vaccine mandate rules to the Supreme Court to test their constitutionality. Between February and March, I was called as an expert (together with some medical scientists and biologists) to reply to the Ministry of Health's statements regarding the vaccines (esp. Pfizer's) in the most prestigious ongoing legal trial, in which a high court was pondering whether to refer the case to the Constitutional Court supporting the unconstitutionality of the obligation. I was called as an ethical and legal expert regarding the licensing procedures and the rules involved and was able to work in full harmony with an extraordinary interdisciplinary team of researchers from all relevant disciplines (medicine, biology, epidemiology, and the like). We had to work day and night for about three weeks to produce a two to three-hundred-page expert report which included not only the legal ethical analysis, but all the relevant scientific updates on the so-called "vaccines." This phase of the trial went well. That high court referred the case to the Constitutional Court, which, in turn, scheduled a decision initially for June and then for the end of November. This upcoming decision will also address the objections of unconstitutionality raised by other judges, and it will be highly dependent on the evolution of "vaccine science" and of the legal debate on relevant constitutional principles and rights.

COVID-19: cosa dicono i fatti," pp. 45-66; S. Gandini, "COVID19: sindemia, misure di prevenzione e rischi per i bambini," pp. 67-78; and A. Donzelli, G. Di Palmo, "Prove di aumento di infezione e di mortalità generale a seguito della vaccinazione," pp. 79-122.

Thus, with some regret, I put aside the English version of this book (which was two-thirds completed) and concentrated—together with the interdisciplinary research groups with whom I was already working —on the actions necessary to facilitate a Constitutional Court's decision based on justice and truth. We have organized, promoted, or facilitated conferences and interviews on a weekly basis all around the country. Above all, from our perspective as scholars, we had to show serious studies and evidence to the Courts. I took on the burden of putting together and editing the relevant publications that had to include, first and foremost, medical scientific updates and sound legal arguments.

In May, a first book edited by me was published which included an authoritative scientific component and a juridical and ethical one. Its title (*Pandemic: An Invitation to Discussion*)[3] came from the title of a conference held in Rome in a hotel next to the Parliament to which we had invited government experts for a fruitful exchange of opinions and data. None of them showed up. On the other hand, the police were sent to surround the square, trying to identify all the participants, discouraging participation, illegitimately pretending to check for vaccine passports, and asking for what reason individuals were walking through the square, which, of course, was deserted. There were only those few people going to the convention building. I was stopped and told the place was dangerous. I asked why, and after some insistence, I was told it was due to a conference. I said that I was one of the speakers, after which they told me that I could pass, then, but I had to show them my "green pass." I replied that I would not show it to them but, if they officially confirmed that the place was dangerous, I would check out from the hotel and go somewhere else. They then told me there was no reason to be alarmed, that I could go safely to the conference. "But you told me it was

3 F. Di Blasi (ed), *Pandemia: Invito al confronto* (Phronesis Publisher: Palermo, 2022).

dangerous," I replied, and I tried for a while longer to carry on that nonsensical discussion, to see if they would finally be honest, admitting that they were just trying to sabotage a conference that the Government did not like. I expected too much of those policemen, who were perhaps even embarrassed by the lies and by that display of patrolling for a conference of scholars. Finally, I left those poor servants of the regime and went to the conference hall where the truth and not regime propaganda would prevail that day.

After May, we had a few other major interdisciplinary conferences and a bigger, more updated book was needed. This time, I had to get additional prominent legal scholars and professionals involved, and I had to do it quickly, because this would truly be helpful if published before November. So, I edited a great new book in which several constitutional lawyers and even a couple of judges from the Italian Supreme Court of Cassation (the highest court of appeal in Italy) joined ethical experts and medical scientists to provide a strong case against the vaccine mandate.[4]

It was only after finishing this new book—after clearing my conscience that I had done everything I could, as a scholar, in this battle of good versus evil—that I made time to complete the English translation of *Vaccination as an act of love?*

This book is very close to my heart, both for the essential truths it conveys in terms of epistemological and ethical principles and for what it means to people like me who suffered persecution just for trying to figure out in good conscience what was best to do for themselves, their families, their churches, and their countries. Yet many things (good and bad) have happened and are still happening since I wrote it, and which I have addressed, for example, in the subsequent edited books just mentioned.[5]

---

4 F. Di Blasi (ed.), *Vaccinazioni COVID-19 e Costituzione: evidenza scientifica e analisi etico-giuridica*, already cited.

5 See also, among my articles already in English, "The US CDC Lies About Myocarditis and Pericarditis," *MedEthica* 1/2022,

(continued on the next page)

On September 19, presumably the same handlers who told Biden that there was a pandemic (which he never understood at all) must have suggested to him that it was over. Today, more and more judges all around the world recognize the absurdities of the pandemic measures.[6] On the negative side, other questionable "vaccines" and/or drugs have been approved and/or authorized.[7] In Europe, for example, the *European Medicines Agency* (EMA) recommended in September final approval of the Pfizer and Moderna "vaccines," which were then approved by the European

---

https://www.questionidibioetica.it/the-us-cdc-lies-about-myocarditis-and-pericarditis/; "Should Unvaccinated People Be Allowed to Get Organ Transplants? A Reply to Arthur L. Caplan," *Questioni di bioetica* 1/2022, https://www.questionidibioetica.it/should-unvaccinated-people-be-allowed-to-get-organ-transplants/; "Mathematical Fraud: The Diabolical Motive Behind Vaccinating Children," *The Postil Magazine*, March 2022, https://www.thepostil.com/mathematical-fraud-the-diabolical-motive-behind-vaccinating-children/?utm_source=sendfox&utm_medium=email&utm_campaign=the-postil-march-newsletter.

6 In the US, see, e.g., A. Katersky, "NYC's COVID vaccine mandate for municipal workers was 'arbitrary and capricious,' judge says," *abc News*, October 26, 2022, https://abcnews.go.com/US/nycs-covid-vaccine-mandate-municipal-workers-arbitrary-capricious/story?id=92086236; J. Musto, "New York judge rules COVID vaccine mandate for NYPD union members invalid," *Fox News*, September 24, 2022, https://www.foxnews.com/health/new-york-judge-rules-covid-vaccine-mandate-nypd-union-members-invalid; J. Q. Nelson, "Federal judge strikes down federal school mask and vaccine mandate for Head Start program," *Fox News*, September 21, 2022, https://www.foxnews.com/media/federal-judge-strikes-down-federal-school-mask-and-vaccine-mandate-head-state-program.

7 See, e.g., F. Di Blasi, "Publication Planning, Early Treatments, and New Super Pills," *Questioni di bioetica*, 1/2022, https://www.questionidibioetica.it/publication-planning-early-treatments-and-new-super-pills/.

Commission, thereby increasing public distrust of health authorities.[8]

There is no way I can even list here the major updates and new important events from the last few months, but I also think that there is no reason to try to write a different book instead of just publishing this English version of the original one. Readers will be perfectly able to find news and updates by themselves, yet they will also profit from the ethical and epistemological points I make in this work, which as such stand on their own. Furthermore, I hope to make my most recent works on the subject available in English very soon as well.

Fulvio Di Blasi

Palermo, October 31, 2022

May Saint Lucilla of Rome, who was blind from birth and recovered her sight at her baptism thanks to her father's faith, help everyone regain their sight and see the truths that were lost during the pandemic

8 I explain and criticize this recommendation and approval in my "Il carattere sperimentale dei vaccini," in F. Di Blasi (ed.), *Vaccinazioni COVID-19 e Costituzione: evidenza scientifica e analisi etico-giuridica*, already cited, pp. 179-184.

Introduction

This book has a structural flaw for which I immediately ask the indulgence of readers, especially fellow philosophers. It concerns the motivation that has finally led me to write it, and that affects mildly the choice of style and bibliographic references of the first two chapters. This defect, however, could at the same time be a virtue for Catholic or, more generally, Christian readers. Let me explain, starting with the motivation.

I. From the Pandemic to this Book

Since the pandemic began, I have resigned myself like everyone else to everything we all had to resign ourselves to. The first lockdown, the second lockdown, curfews, masks, hand sanitizers, work and family difficulties, the rules for going to Mass and to the supermarket, the abolition of travel and holidays, the new waves, the hopes for vaccines that, perhaps, would save us; and, again, the economic crisis, the monopolization of existential and mass media news, focused every day on the bulletin of deaths and infections, on new outbreaks, on new yellow or red areas, on the latest rules to follow, on the reactions of individual states, but also on some new TV show personalities, especially virologists and epidemiologists or those presumed to be such.

I've become familiar with things that I almost didn't know existed before, at least from an existential point of view, but which have forcefully entered my daily sources of interest and information. Things like drug agencies, the World Health Organization, their protocols and conflicts of interest, emergency approval procedures, journals, and university departments of medicine. I reluctantly agreed to read and discuss all these things every day in social networks. I have also lived through new experiences of which I have a positive or still uncertain balance.

My young children have had contact with their parents that few children have ever had in our busy world. My baby girl was born just before the first lockdown. Thank God, we had just managed to repair the house from serious mold problems and to return there between the end of January and February 2020. I and my wife, who is also a lawyer and scholar passionate about culture and everything else, had never imagined spending such long periods of monastic isolation, work, and intimacy.

We too, at home, have had our *waves* and *regulatory* changes. There was that of pizza and homemade desserts. There was that of sports played with children on the terrace (also to work off sweets and pizza). There was that of the camping on the terrace, where we set up a large family tent on an artificial lawn for Christmas 2020, surrounded by solar-powered Christmas lights (the holiday budget was spent in 2020, and with better results, in this way). There was that of the giant terrace nativity scene, with water pump and waterfalls and real ornamental plants, built at home with the children by carving and painting polystyrene and wooden boards for the stable. There have been attempts at homeschooling, also with the help of heroic grandparents who have come over as much as possible, despite the curfews and occasional swab tests, also to allow us to isolate ourselves from time to time in a room to get some work done. There have been such beautiful and genuine family experiences that, at times, with my wife, we even were thankful for the pandemic, roughly with that spirit with which, in the Easter Mass, since St. Augustine, we refer to original sin in terms of *felix culpa*.

Smart working and the development of new online work options are certainly among the positive aspects of the epidemic. Today we have learned more about how many things can be done remotely with the technologies we have available. Smart or remote working allows many people, in many ways, to better reconcile their professional life with their personal and family life. Let's hope there is no turning back in this area, after the emergency is over.

I think back on all this, not without ardor, to say that, even in the worst moments of the pandemic, I had never thought of making a professional effort to talk about it. Even when, taking seriously some of my wife's perplexities, I had a second thought about vaccines and government policies, and when I began to study relevant sources of information with greater professional attention and to listen to online lectures and specialized conferences on the subject, I didn't think even for a moment of writing a book about it. Even when the witch hunt against the so-called anti-vaxxers began, when the mass media and politics started to treat me, my wife, and many of our friends and colleagues who had doubts about vaccines and about the decisions to be made about them as if we were fools and idiots to mock and publicly insult.... Even in this predicament I didn't think about writing a book on the subject. In fact, my initial reaction was the opposite. I decided to stop reading many newspapers or watching television and instead to concentrate on other books I was writing. Unfortunately, hateful excerpts of pseudo-journalistic talk shows conducted in the name of ignorance, arrogance and insult still tormented me through the clips that inevitably populated social media. Still, not even this additional pressure incited me to the point of turning everything I had studied and found out about the pandemic into a book. Posting some occasional ironic, outraged, or staggered comments on social media was enough to distract me so I could let it out and go back to my regular work.

There was one thing that broke the camel's back, though, and it was not about my professional life but about my life of faith. Political institutions had breached their fundamental duty to respect the truth and freedom of their citizens. They violated the right of every free person to receive correct and honest information. They had tried demagogically to bend and control people's will, intelligence, and conduct. Physicians, after the first wave of heroism, so charged with magnanimity and exemplarity, had finally allowed themselves to be harnessed and standardized downwards by a political power that wanted them to be bureaucrats who stayed far away from patients, at least until hospitalizations. They had allowed themselves to be replaced by sloppy and generic directives from impersonal government agencies, reduced to paper pushing, thus mortifying the exercise of a profession that always begins and ends with care and attention for the patient. Scientists had also failed by letting a generic, magical, and mystical reference to a higher and nonexistent entity called "Science" take the place—in the common feeling and in the demagogy of ignorant and unscrupulous politicians and journalists—of serious and real discussion among scholars and of critical thinking. Journalism had died, replaced by the will to power of those who have the media in their hands and decide to use the media only and exclusively to convince everyone of their prejudices and to make the masses conform to the decisions of the political class. But shouldn't journalism be the bulwark of investigation and real democracy precisely in times when politics risks having too much free rein and too much power?

Yet, despite everything, despite all these failures, it was still enough for me to turn off the TV, close the online pages of the new regime's newspapers, and concentrate on my family, my research, and my books.

One thing, as I said, finally stopped me from simply closing the door and staying at home doing my own thing: the failure of the church. I am referring, of course, not to the true Church, that is, to the Mystical Body of Christ, which lives in the mystery of His People, and which walks in history assisted by the Spirit of Truth. The true Church is the humanity of Christ, God incarnate who becomes a sacrament, who becomes the mystery of God's presence among us. When God becomes man, matter becomes direct contact with the supernatural: "Philip said to him, "Master, show us the Father, and that will be enough for us." Jesus said to him, "Have I been with you for so long a time and you still do not know me, Philip? Whoever has seen me has seen the Father. How can you say, 'Show us the Father'?" (John 14: 9-10).

The Incarnation does not end with the ascension of Jesus into Heaven. The Incarnation remains until the end of time. It's just that, after the Ascension, the sacramental mystery doubles. While two thousand years ago, we saw Jesus and, by touching His humanity, we really and mysteriously touched God, now we don't see Him, but we really and mysteriously touch God by touching His sacramental humanity, which is truly present in His People. Whoever does not understand that the Church is the Body of Christ incarnate which continues to walk and act mysteriously in history with the legs and arms of His faithful has not understood anything significant about the Church. This Church, for a believer, can never fail. Men, however, are fallible and sinful. Even the righteous sins seven times a day, which is an important warning against any presumption and idolatry of personalities. Here on earth, no one is holy, and we all must always be very careful. Only the People of God as a whole are Holy, because they are the Body of Christ.

The church as a human institution is made up of men who are all fallible, starting with the Pope (except of course for those very rare times in history in which he speaks ex cathedra on matters of faith and morals). The Church as a militant People (that is, without considering those in Purgatory and Paradise) is made up of three types of faithful, all called to be saints in the same way and all cells of the Mystical Body of Christ: there are clerics (deacons, priests, and bishops), there are the religious (who make vows and who could also be clerics at the same time), and there are the lay faithful. Nobody is in the big-league team, and nobody is in little, or very little, leagues. The dignity of every believer is rooted in the call to communion with God and in letting Christ work in him to impact the history of the world. Clerics have an institutional responsibility, but if some or many clerics make a mistake, Christ will work more through other faithful, because the true, sacramental Church is never in the hands of any single person or group of mere men.

When I talk about the failure of the church in these times of pandemic, I am therefore referring to the failure of many clerics (not all, thank God), who should be talking about the saving message of the Gospel and the truths revealed by God and who instead talk about vaccines and of the green pass as if these things belonged to the *depositum fidei*. I speak of the failure of a church that generates ethical doubts about things that belong to the conscience and prudential reasoning of every faithful individual. I am speaking of a church that aligns and allies itself with political or economic power, mistaking its supernatural ministry for assistance to the dubious or questionable policies of the rulers of the moment. I speak of a church that remains silent in the face of demagogy and disinformation. I speak of a church indifferent to the persecution of so many righteous. I am speaking of a church that discriminates and generates conflicts among its own faithful for the benefit of the transitional policies of utilitarian rulers. I'm talking about a church that has turned its priorities and value hierarchies upside-down. Where are the atheists and anti-Catholics, who always scream at alleged medieval obscurantism, in these days when spiritual power and temporal power seem to inexplicably walk hand in hand?

When the "churchmen" praise politicians too much or rejoice too much in their attention or seek them too much or manifest too many inferiority complexes with respect to political institutions or no longer know how to distinguish the freedoms of the Church from the freedoms of politics, I become particularly worried. Clerics are no more intelligent than the lay faithful. It is often the other way around. And this is the reason why they make themselves so often ridiculous with the politicians and the powerful on duty. Many clerics have an inferiority complex because they do not feel equal to the world. Economics, politics, and science are too high for them, too unreachable, and, without realizing it, they end up kneeling facing the wrong way, no longer in the direction of the Altar. We lay people do not have these problems. We are the politicians, the scientists, and the economists. We cannot have any inferiority complex towards ourselves. And I am convinced that it is also for this reason that, in times like the present ones, in which the church of clerics is the victim of its own inferiority complexes and generates too much confusion and division among the faithful, the Mystical Body tends to inspire the laity more to the responsibility of distinguishing the boundaries of the *depositum fidei*, on the one hand, and of what belongs to Caesar, on the other.

The straw that broke the camel's back, and that led me to this book, was hearing the greatest religious authority in the world say that getting vaccinated is an act of love, thus providing an assist to the political authorities who sought to proclaim that vaccination is a civic duty. At this point, the poor faithful Catholic who has doubts about the vaccine, and that he is also a good citizen, is surrounded. Is his doubt then an act of selfishness? Is it a temptation from the devil? Is it an act contrary to the common good? In addition to his own religious and political authority, he is at the same time discriminated against and persecuted by all with the complicity of the mainstream media. He has become the villain to be ridiculed as the selfish enemy of the common good, with the blessing of the Pope and the Presidents. All this is unacceptable and, in my own little way, it required me to at least put my professional skills to use in the service of the persecuted righteous

II. The Structural Defect (or Virtue)

I explained the motivation. Let's go back to the defect. This book is an essay on applied ethics that requires the use of conceptual technical tools that mainly concern the theory of action and epistemology. In what follows, I have to face the problem of a moral choice that potentially has the vaccine against Covid as its object. Yet, I cannot, of course, fully address all the questions of fundamental ethics that are the prerequisite for an analysis of the human act.

You cannot write a textbook on moral philosophy every time you have to deal with a specific moral issue in detail. Still, the reader must be offered an understandable summary of the most important tools to use. I cannot explain how nails and hammers are made, but I must at least make these tools available to the reader. All it takes is a simple introduction, as short as possible, to be able to immediately get into the topic and open the construction site.

For the purposes of this book, I will almost exclusively use simple philosophical tools which are now part of the shared cultural heritage of Western civilization and which, to a large extent, have been institutionalized through law. Aristotle had already begun, in the third book of his *Nicomachean Ethics*, to analyze the meaning and characteristics of the voluntary act as a prerequisite for moral action. Today, when we discuss liability in civil or criminal courtrooms, we take for granted that we must, on the one hand, identify a certain human act, lawful or unlawful (the contract of sale, for example, or the crime of theft), and, on the other hand, analyze its voluntariness: that is, understand how and to what extent that act can be traced back to the psychic sphere of the person who, allegedly, performed it.

The first operation is, in a certain sense, objective or material; the second is subjective (related to the subject). We may be faced with a document that looks like a contract, but which is void because it was not freely signed. We may have a case of murder before us, but it is not really such because the perpetrator was under the influence of drugs and was induced by third parties. Perhaps, however, the murderer was partly aware and consenting. The effect of the drugs could then function as a mitigating circumstance. However, it could be an aggravating circumstance that he killed with particular brutality. This aspect of brutality would then comply with the objective analysis of what happened, but it would also affect the assessment of the criminal's subjective responsibility.

All this can be summarized by saying that, when studying a human act, it is necessary to carry out both an objective analysis of the moral act that includes all the relevant circumstances, and an analysis of the agent's intentionality, which basically consists of two things: the knowledge he had of what he was about to do (the intellectual aspect of the moral choice) and the voluntariness with which he chose what his intellect offered him as a possibility (the willful aspect of the moral act). Knowledge and voluntariness: these are the two primary concepts of subjective responsibility. There is no freedom without knowledge of what one does and without intentionality and voluntary choice.

Now, if we were to discuss fundamental ethics, or even legal theory, each of these elements could be problematized indefinitely. What is the boundary between the material description of the deed and the choice of it? How are material and psychological causation determined? How does the appetite for the purpose determine the choice? How do you pass from universal knowledge to the knowledge of an action? What is the relationship between virtue and the rule of action? What makes the subject truly free, good, or vicious? Moral philosophers and jurists quickly understand how fascinating and inexhaustible these questions are. Each of these aspects may require more than one book. The macroscopic tools of analysis, however, can be shared even by philosophers and jurists of very distant or even opposing backgrounds. It is at this level of sharing that they are routinely used in courts and in public ethical, legal, and political debate.

It is at this level of sharing that the basic concepts of this book are placed, forming the background for the analysis of applied ethics that I propose to undertake. This analysis, in its basic structure, and independently from the terminology used (which at times the reader might like more or less), can therefore be shared by anyone regardless of philosophical differences on the themes of fundamental ethics or the theory of law. Still, the problem remains of how to explain these basic tools and concepts to the reader. How am I supposed to get the nails and the hammer into his hands? Probably, if I had chosen to write this book at the beginning of the year, I would have done so mainly using Aristotle, or, as mentioned above, our shared instruments of Western law. If I had chosen to write a book on the same topic but unrelated to public debate, I would probably have set the basic theoretical discourse using Thomas Aquinas, who is my favorite author and about whom, as a scholar, I am more of an expert.

As I said before, however, the ultimate motivation for this book came from the unjust attack that I believe I suffered, together with many friends, especially as a Catholic from other Catholics. Therefore, it came naturally to me to supply nails and hammer to the reader in the simplest possible way in which I would have given them to any Catholic: that is to say, on the basis of the traditional teaching of the Church on moral conscience and on the sources of the morality of human acts (a teaching, by the way, which has always developed in parallel with Roman law and Western philosophy). Anti-Catholic or atheist philosophers will have to forgive me for this approach in the first two introductory chapters and will have to be able to look beyond it. The analysis of applied ethics within the book does not depend in itself on Catholic thought, but uses it as an example of some shared ethical tools and as a contextualization of my personal motivations. I must say, in any case, that reading some Catholic references to these issues, especially with respect to conscience, can be culturally beautiful even for those who are not Catholics or Christians, even for those who are atheists. Those who are open to culture always appreciate it, even when they don't share in it. Above all, they appreciate those who are honest about their preferred cultural and bibliographic references.

Let me return for a moment to the intellectual aspect of ethical choice, or to knowing what you choose. This aspect makes us appreciate why epistemology is so important in this book. In fact, in order to understand how to behave with respect to vaccines and the pandemic, it is necessary to understand exactly the truth value of the information we have about them. First, we need to know what our actual options are; then, we can freely and responsibly decide what it is best to do. In this field, however, the options depend on a lot of information that comes from many people and from different disciplines such as medicine, epidemiology, biology, law, and ethics. Within each of these disciplines we must be able to evaluate the meaning and value of the information that is provided to us. From this point of view, epistemological analysis is the necessary premise of ethical analysis in a book such as this one.

III. The Scientific Character of this Work

This is a book on ethical theory, and it is important to understand its scope and methodology from the outset. Ethics is the area to which the choices of the individual or the political community belong. Ethics is the science that tries to determine the criteria of goodness or badness of human actions. In the actions necessary for coexistence with others, goodness is called justice. The first treatise on justice in history is found in Aristotle's ethics, as it is among the virtues that the *phronimos*, or the good and just man, ought to embody. Aristotle's politics is a continuation of his ethics. Politics is that part of ethical science that has collective common action as its object instead of individual action. A law or a sentence are human actions whose goodness is called justice. In this book, I adopt a classic approach according to which law is part of ethics, that part that concerns the goodness of the actions necessary for civil coexistence.

I state this premise for several reasons. One is so that my reader will have to learn to recognize the ethical or legal nature of certain decisions, because both their epistemology and the correct analysis of the reasoning that justifies them depend on this. There is enormous confusion about these things. Some, for example, may think that the decision of an agency such as the Food and Drug Administration (FDA) to authorize the use of a vaccine is of a medical or scientific nature. Nothing could be more wrong. Others may think that choosing to get vaccinated is not an ethical choice. This is also wrong.

The debate that has taken place over the past two years is schizophrenic because it constantly refers to an alleged and unspecified "*Science*" to justify decisions that are fundamentally ethical and juridical. Then, when experts in moral philosophy or law try to clarify some essential aspects of those decisions, they are treated as if they were incompetent, when instead there are too many alleged scientists who practice ethics and law without realizing it and without having the competence to do so. This book is a text on individual and political ethics that also aims to reestablish the proper boundaries between the respective skills of each of the experts involved in the current pandemic crisis.

Many fellow moral philosophers will disagree with me in considering law as part of ethics. So be it! Still, they underestimate a very important aspect of law that they should rather learn to exploit in order to be more analytical and precise. In fact, the law forces precision because it requires shared ethical reasoning for the purposes of public decision making. The natural development of Aristotelian theory of action is to be found in the manuals of private law and criminal law, where one finds the fine details of how to identify a human action and how to evaluate its subjective and intentional aspects. The moral philosopher can afford little precision in the classroom where he lectures, but when he enters court as a lawyer, a single small inaccuracy can cost him the case. An analysis of legal reasoning seeks to shed painstaking clarity on which facts and concepts may justify a certain decision. A judge's verdict is the perfect laboratory animal to use for studying the moral reasoning that justifies a certain choice or decision. In the judge's sentence, that reasoning must appear in all its premises and logical sequences. A substantial and essential part of this book will make use, for example, of the science regarding witnesses, of which legal science is the expert and which too many people underestimate while using it continuously to support their moral and political choices.

Some colleagues are free to think that law is not part of ethics, and this will not detract from their reading and potential appreciation of my work. Yet I invite them to reflect on the fact that law is the place where the rules of behavior, on the one hand, and reasoning on action, on the other, must necessarily find a shared meeting point. This has advantages and disadvantages. Shared solutions are not always the best or the most rational. However, when everyone has to discuss them in an open and verifiable way in view of a necessary decision (the verdict), the bar is raised. If some moral philosophers were forced to present their theses in the scientific context of a courtroom, they would learn to argue them better, and many eccentric and imaginative ideas would be exposed and rejected (probably by the authors themselves).

Lawyers are not moral philosophers. Jurists use ethics in a qualified way, through scientific and systematic knowledge of the rules shared by society and the reasoning that led to their application. Consequently, they have a natural familiarity with moral reasoning and a natural passion for discussions of fundamental ethics. Moral philosophers, for their part, are not jurists and, not being limited by shared norms or by their application, they can question their ultimate foundations and presuppositions. From jurists, however, they can learn how to really work with norms and how to think about concrete human actions. While the philosopher doubts the very possibility of moral responsibility, the jurist must decide whether a certain person should go to prison. The first doubt is legitimate in fundamental ethical theory, but not knowing how to resolve the second question is a lacuna both in fundamental ethical theory and in the analysis of the moral act.

Another advantage of the jurist over the (mere) moral philosopher is that the first is very familiar with experts and expert opinions. A good lawyer needs to figure out which technical consultants he needs for a certain case, be it an engineer, a doctor, an epidemiologist, or a nuclear physicist. A good judge can read the reports and make his decision. For this reason, it is said, in jargon, that the judge is *peritus peritorum*, the expert on experts. A similar thing happens at the political level when a parliament needs to listen to experts on a certain subject. However good the experts are, even the parliament remains *peritus peritorum*, because parliament decides on the basis of the common good and not of the good of a single discipline. This does not mean that technical advice cannot be essential to a certain political or judicial decision. It only means that the jurist must be an expert epistemologist, capable of evaluating the exact probative value of a certain piece of technical advice. What exactly is this doctor's expertise telling me about the murder case? What exactly does this scientist tell me about the common good? What exactly does this virologist tell me about the advisability of urgently authorizing a vaccine or making it mandatory? Even in these cases, legal experience can help also those moral philosophers who believe that law is different from morality. For the purposes of this book, I'd be fine calling them cousins instead of brothers, as long as we understand that law and morals are both essential and intertwined with each other.

This is an ethics book on Covid vaccines and the pandemic. Ethics, like law, requires trained technical consultants on all issues involved in certain decisions. In this text, therefore, doctors, virologists, biologists, epidemiologists, statisticians, etc. have a decisive role. They play a decisive role because an ethical decision cannot be made without awareness of all the relevant factors. It is an epistemological error, however, to think that the final competence on moral choice can be reduced to the specific competences of individual consultants, just as how a judge's verdict cannot be reduced to the expert opinions filed by lawyers, or how the law of a parliament cannot be reduced to the opinions of the experts who testified during the preparatory stages.

This is an ethics book on vaccines that does not intend to give a definitive ethical answer because such an answer, in this case, does not exist and because any prudent answer ultimately belongs to all those, individuals or authorities, who have to decide how to act. The moral philosopher can only help to highlight the logical presuppositions of the choice and the factors to consider. And this is no small thing, because knowledge makes you free.

IV. My Scientific and Intellectual Conversions

I too have been a victim of the propaganda of these two years, and I have discovered that I had always lived in a worrying sleep of reason with respect to other basic themes and issues that the pandemic has now brought powerfully to the attention of the world. Initially, I was very confident that, despite the virus having taken the world off guard, the right decisions were being made at the global political level.

I was initially a big proponent of lockdown and was amazed at the approaches of Sweden or the UK. I thought it was essential to make the new vaccines immediately available to African and other poor countries. I was convinced that vaccines were the only way to get out of the pandemic and that we should focus fully on walking the vaccine path. I had never seriously doubted bodies such as the Food and Drug Administration (FDA), the European Medicines Agency (EMA), which I hardly knew existed, or the World Health Organization (WHO).

Then I had some doubts and started studying. As always, serious study does not lead to dogmatism, fanaticism, or easy certainties. Rather, it brings other more significant doubts that become precious for progress and for better and more prudent choices at all levels. In many areas of knowledge, studying will never eliminate the risks of decisions, but it will allow us to better evaluate them and to understand if, when, and how to make them.

Today, I believe that the generalized lockdown was a mistake in many states, and that it is certainly not the right choice for others. I think politicians should understand much better how this tool is tailored to the specificities of each political community. I believe that drug agencies are corroded and limited by serious situations of conflict of interest, lack of professional competence, and lack of independence whose solution is not at all easy, but really urgent. I believe that too many and serious mistakes have been made on the new vaccines and that a change of course is urgently needed, even with respect to vaccination in the poorest countries where there is no evidence of pandemic emergency. I believe that many aspects of the democratic order have been undervalued and that the consequences are already being felt.

What I mean here, in a nutshell, is that by studying we change our mind; things become problematic, and that's a good thing. Never be afraid of people thinking and posing questions. One of the biggest mistakes of many world political authorities and too many journalists has been to set their action on indoctrinating citizens rather than on informing them with sincerity and on trusting them, on using carrots and sticks rather than reasoning and calls to responsibility and patriotism. It is never too late, though, and this is also one of the hopes that prompted me to commit myself to this job. In the long run (and, sometimes, hopefully, even in the short and medium ones), the world belongs to those who decide to be smart and take action.

V. Not a Book on Vaccines

I have to make it clear right away that this is not a book about vaccines. This is a very important clarification to be made to avoid misunderstandings. In fact, one of the most demagogic and sophistical strategies used by the new regime of politics, journalism, and religion's unified thought has been to create this surreal contrast between people who are supposedly in favor of vaccines and people who are supposedly against vaccines.

I do not want to emphasize that this contrast is not real. This is a sufficiently obvious point to which, in any case, I will return often and from various angles in the course of my discussion. No, here I want to say something different and extremely important for a scholar who approaches his object of study with sufficient detachment and scientificity. I cannot simply assume that the so-called anti-Covid vaccines that we are using around the world in emergency mode are definable as vaccines. Maybe they are, maybe not.

The starting scientific data is that until last year, these new products of the pharmaceutical industry, made with technologies never used before and about which little is known, would not have been defined as vaccines. A serious scholar cannot therefore assume that they are. This is something I'll come back to in more detail later, of course, but it was certainly a technical mistake to advertise them and present them to the world as vaccines. Why? It's obvious. Vaccines are a type of drug with respect to which a great deal of promotion activity has rightly been done for years to facilitate their acceptance and understanding by the population. There has been a huge effort to create an environment of worldwide scientific trust around vaccines. The term 'vaccine' was until yesterday for medicine like the phrase 'Made in Italy' was for fashion and food. There was serious and well-founded trust in this brand.

It is obvious that any manufacturer of clothes or food would sell their mother if, for some emergency reason, they had the possibility of obtaining the 'Made in Italy' label on their own new product. It is obvious that being able to use the 'vaccine' brand for a new product is like striking gold for pharmaceutical companies, which may even lead to the market of mandatory pharmacological uses. We should have been very careful, though, because if this new product doesn't really behave as a vaccine or if it generates distrust in vaccines, years of excellent work spent on building a reliable, successful brand will be thrown into the trash. A bit like if the worst or the most hated and contested dress in the world had been produced with the 'Made in Italy' brand. Calling these new products 'vaccines' has not been scientifically accurate or prudent. Sure, it was the biggest and most clever marketing operation that pharmaceutical companies could do, but it was done to the detriment of medicine and public trust. One can only hope that things will eventually turn out well. It was a mistake, though. I have no doubts about this, and it is one of those things that I have discovered, and of which I am now convinced, by studying, not from initial prejudices. And that's the only way, by studying, that I expect other serious people to possibly disagree with me.

In my discussion, I will often refer to these products as 'vaccines' for mere convenience, as they are talked about like this. Sometimes, I will refer to them differently to remind the reader that they do not necessarily deserve this name and that it is still a brand name that, for them, is, at least for those who understand it, *sub iudice*.

VI. Data that Changes Continuously

As I said earlier, this is an ethics book that requires a lot of scientific data and knowledge, which I have obviously learned from experts in the relevant fields. One of the problems with the data and scientific knowledge about Covid vaccines, however, is that they change all the time. There are literally many updates and new data to be monitored and considered daily.

Obviously, this type of work concerns me only in a marginal or tangential way because I, in fact, do not write about medicine, statistics, or biology. It is not my job to constantly update the population on technical and scientific data. I try to take due account, as far as possible, of any relevant updates up to the time of publication. Then, however, this type of activity will become the concern of every reader, who will need to check many other more direct and qualified sources.

My relationship with the updating of data and news must be evaluated with respect to my scientific field, which is the ethical, legal, and epistemological one. What a book like this can do is clarify how to interpret data from various sources and disciplines in order to form one's own judgment of conscience on vaccines and, in general, on the pandemic. Again, this book can help to identify the main relevant sources. It can help to understand how to identify and evaluate the relevant criteria for moral choice. Then, once the structure of ethical reasoning is well constructed and outlined, everyone will be able to update its content with the new data available to them.

The same thing happened to me too because, in fact, this book was not born from prejudice, but from a serious and detailed effort to clarify first to myself how to interpret the times in which we are living with respect to choices regarding vaccines and the pandemic emergency. Thus, it happened to me that, after a certain level of analysis in which I was able to insert data and knowledge in appropriate categories and specific chapters, it became very easy for me to quickly update myself on the news of the day in order to evaluate the current status of my choices. Indeed, as I will clarify in the first part of the work, the ethical choice on these issues is not made once and for all, but must instead be constantly updated in a diachronic sense—all the more reason to shy away from any categorical labels, such as anti-vaxxers, pro-vaxxers, vaccine fanatics, etc.

VII. The Architecture of this Work

The ethical structure of this work has always been clear to me from the very beginning. After a brief introduction on the structure and evaluation criteria of the moral act, I would focus on these new vaccines as an object of ethical or political choice. I would therefore analyze them according to the fundamental concepts of the object, circumstances, and the end. This analysis would highlight all possible levels of criticality, doubts, certainties, and uncertainties with respect to each of these concepts and with respect to the overall ethical evaluation of the choice.

However, problems arose in the transition from fundamental ethics to applied ethics: that is, when sufficiently identifying the "anti-Covid vaccine" object with respect to the essential circumstances of this object and the possible ends of choosing it. This type of analysis required me to make constant systematic and conceptual changes regarding the various elements involved: changes that were sometimes so significant that a chapter jumped from one part of the work to another or grew into two, three, five chapters or into one entire part of the overall work. Thus, from an initial hypothesis of division into chapters, I finally moved on to a book consisting of several parts, each of which was divided into chapters.

However, the work had reached dimensions that I had not initially imagined. And, even while skipping and avoiding many interesting but non-essential topics, I found that my preparation time was getting longer and longer. But I wanted the book to be useful, especially in these weeks and months of great uncertainty and tension. Indeed, I was not motivated by a mere theoretical objective, but by an ethical one. I wanted to help and support individual and collective choices, as well as to assist with the debate concerning these choices. Each day of delay was a failure for me. I therefore decided to divide the work into several volumes. This would allow me to start publishing it while I was still working on refining and completing its various parts.

Consider that the first volume (which includes the first two parts of the work) required a full month just for the correction and editing of the Italian and English versions. A month may seem long to some, but it is a very short review period for a scholarly book. Normally, reviewers take at least a few weeks to read it and send appropriate considerations, corrections, suggestions, etc. Then, it takes a few weeks to take these recommendations into consideration with due attention, and a few extra weeks to evaluate how they came up against the reviewers' recommendations. Then, again, there are the editorial drafts to be corrected with the publishing house. If I hadn't divided the work into several volumes, I would probably not have been able to make it available before June 2022. In this way, however, I should be able to publish the various volumes more or less monthly starting in December 2021. This is a great advantage for the scientific debate and for all the friends who constantly ask me to give them my qualified opinion on the subject as soon as possible.

With this premise, let me now lay out the plan or architecture of the parts of the work.

Part I: The Structure of the Moral Act

In this part of the work, I expose the fundamental conceptual tools with which it is possible to analyze and evaluate the moral act. I dwell above all on moral conscience, on ethical choice, and on the concepts of object, circumstances, and end. I also set out my principles and criteria of analysis, my relationship with the sources, and the definitional difficulties relating to the object "vaccine" and to the circumstances that may surround the choice of it.

Part II: Internal Structural Institutional Circumstances

In this part of the work, I deal with the intrinsic circumstances of the anti-Covid vaccines that characterize their regulatory framework: that is, the way in which the object "anti-Covid vaccine" exists as a choice in the legal system. More specifically, among these circumstances, I address those that precede the specific application criteria for vaccines. In this same part of the book, I also set out the main epistemological criteria of my analysis.

Part III: Selective and Evaluative Internal Institutional Circumstances

In this part of the work, I deal with the intrinsic circumstances of anti-Covid vaccines that characterize their regulatory framework, and which specifically concern the administration of vaccines to individuals (based on their medical situation, their age, etc.). This study involves a detailed analysis of the authorization documents of the individual vaccines by the FDA and EMA above all.

Part IV: The Death of Phronimos: Faith and Truth About Vaccines

In this part of the work, I deal with circumstances that do not pertain in themselves to the good of health and to the way in which the vaccine relates as a tool to this good. At the theoretical level, this part presupposes: a) a specific study in theory of knowledge regarding our way of knowing the truth; b) a specific study in virtue ethics aimed at rediscovering the ethical and epistemological criteria to be used to give trust to those who propose certain truths; and c) the analysis of the reliability of the various witnesses of the truth about anti-Covid vaccines, from pharmaceutical companies to public agencies, science, governments and the mass media.[9]

Part V: Internal Non-Institutional Circumstances

In this part of the work, I deal with the intrinsic circumstances of anti-Covid vaccines that can determine the choice to use them or not to use them based on elements and criteria independent of their legal regulation. In this study, the reference sources are no longer government agencies, but above all independent science and medical practice.

Part VI: The Intentionality of the End

In this part of the work, I move from the analysis of the object and the circumstances to that of the purposes of moral action. An important theoretical part of this study concerns the analysis of intentionality, human goods, and so-called subjective morality. Here I also address the issues of the relationship between the person and

9 For editorial reasons, the volume containing this part of the work was published first, with the title, *The Death of the Phronimos: Faith and Truth on Anti-Covid Vaccines* (Phronesis Publisher: Palermo, 2021).

> the common good, and the utilitarianism that predominantly characterizes the current political choices of governments.

This book's acknowledgments echo those of *The Death of the Phronimos*, whose writing essentially took place in parallel.

As always, I thank God for giving me the opportunity to make another small contribution in this world with the time and the talents that have been given to me. I thank my wife Francesca for the patience, support, encouragement, and enthusiasm with which she always deals with the things that concern our cultural commitments for the common good. With respect to the specific issue of anti-Covid vaccines and pandemic management, it was initially she who stimulated my critical approach and prompted me to study the relevant issues more in depth. I also thank my children, Riccardo and Ottavia, because their cheerful presence alone, even if it makes it difficult to concentrate, gives a joy and hope capable of overcoming any obstacle and fatigue. The other day I found Riccardo, five years old, drawing in a notebook while sitting on the sofa; as soon as he saw me, he immediately told me that he too was writing a book. Ottavia (two years old) is at this moment on my lap, between me and the computer, enjoying herself while listening to kids' songs on television and while I stretch my arms around her trying to reach the keyboard and finish this introduction. *Deo gratias*!

I thank my friend Mauro Ghilardini who was one of the immediate causes of this work because, since he decided to publish some of my posts on a blog, so many comments and requests for clarifications or insights followed that it was easier for me to think of writing a book than responding to a thousand posts online. I thank Peter Doshi for his comments, suggestions, and useful discussions and exchanges of ideas. I thank Marisa Gatti-Taylor Ph.D. and Steven Millen Taylor Ph.D.—as well as a friend who needs to remain anonymous to avoid possible negative employment repercussions—for their precious editorial help and for their encouragement. Of course, I am solely responsible for errors and opinions expressed in the text. I thank all the friends, colleagues, physicians, and scientists who maintain rationality, integrity, and serenity in these times of collective panic and madness. I thank all the people of good will who do not give in to violence, insult, and social hatred and who never tire of demonstrating publicly for the protection of the fundamental rights and freedoms of the human person. Finally, I thank all the bishops and priests who continue to preach the Gospel of Christ instead of the new vaccine and Green Pass religion.

Part I

The structure of moral act

This part of the work, as already mentioned in the introduction, is intended to outline for the reader, in the simplest and most immediate way possible, the frame of reference for our ethical analysis of anti-Covid vaccines. The first pieces of the framework are of course moral conscience, the reasoning with which we evaluate how to behave, and the relationship between freedom and the rule of action. From this follow the so-called sources of the morality of human acts: object, circumstances, and the end.

We must become familiar with the ethical legal methodology of observing a human act or a choice from the point of view of the objective and subjective elements that characterize it. The description of the choice is not easy, and often, as we will see, there is no precise boundary between object, circumstances, and end, or between objective and subjective morality. However, many gray areas are of little or no relevance to the overall ethical assessment. The important thing is to give the right weight to each relevant factor.

The last chapter of this part of the text, in addition to distinguishing the points of view from which to identify the circumstances and to classify their possible types, is also an opportunity to explain some basic principles or criteria of analysis, such as the use of the epistemological method and of the legal one, the use of official sources and documents, and the prudent or patient relationship we should always have with the analytical approach to ethics.

Chapter 1

Moral Conscience and the Sources of Morality

In a context in which the subject of the pandemic enjoys a total worldwide media monopoly, a video message from Pope Francis on August 18, 2021, in which he said that "vaccination is an act of love," caused an immediate sensation. Unlike the Gospel of Jesus Christ, this message was not a sign of contradiction for humanity, which rather welcomed it with enormous euphoria, making it immediately go viral in all the media in the world. Indeed, in this case the disciple, regrettably, was greater than his Master.[10]

In the ongoing battle between the so-called pro-vaxxers and anti-vaxxers, where the former enjoy the support of politics and public information while the latter include many ordinary people with ethical doubts about vaccines, the Pope's statement was immediately turned into the perfect weapon against anti-vaxxers. This minority found itself immediately under a siege now blessed by the Pope, and it was insulted and persecuted as never before. The alleged anti-vaxxers (which anti-vaxxers are mostly not, but the label, you know, is an alluring weapon) have

10 "Remember the word I spoke to you, 'No slave is greater than his master.' If they persecuted me, they will also persecute you." (John 15:20).

been defined as selfish, immoral, imbecilic, ignorant, mice to be locked up in their cages, enemies of society, terrorists, people to be tracked down and prosecuted, or to be refused the care and assistance of the national health system, or again, to be taxed, fired, ostracized and even wished a painful and humiliating death, a death which would be liberating for society and for those who, through the vaccine, have performed their *act of love*.

For these persecuted, humiliated, and offended subjects there was no word of comfort from the church, which, if anything, anointed and consecrated their persecutors, thanks to the raising of that personal opinion of the Pope to universal ethical truth. Even many dioceses and parishes have initiated policies of discrimination and humiliation against these 'criminals' (deprived even of due process), limiting their participation in ecclesial activities and even in liturgical celebrations.[11] I myself could recount the bitterness and insults of many churchmen against alleged anti-vaxxers who tried to reason with them. But doesn't Christ stay with those who are persecuted and oppressed? Doesn't Christian ethics lie in the honest reasoning of people of conscience?

For those who have followed the debates on Covid and the vaccines in the media and on social networks, the hatred generated by that statement from the Pope—used, I repeat, as a weapon against the doubters—was so evident as to arouse a surreal impression. For the wiser and more intelligent, the painful rift between ecclesial institutions and the true faith has increased. Is it really possible that a virus was enough to create such confusion between love and hate or between good and evil in the entire

11 On the way in which the Pope's statement created difficulties in obtaining exemption from the vaccine for religious reasons, see P. Gondreau, "COVID Vaccines and the Religious Exemption," *Catholic Answers*, December 03, 2021, URL: https://www.catholic.com/magazine/online-edition/covid-vaccines-and-the-religious-exemption.

Christian and world community? Shouldn't whoever caused so much confusion and so much hatred have immediately intervened on behalf of the oppressed and clarified what true love is? If trees can be recognized by their fruits, these fruits alone are enough to settle the matter. If the idea that getting vaccinated is an act of love causes so much hatred towards those who have doubts about the vaccine, if these are the fruits of this idea, then it is a sign that it must be amended immediately.

At the technical level, however, all this is alien to the hypothetical truthful content of what the Pope affirmed. In other words, it is logically possible that the Pope, who has the primary responsibility of bearing witness to the truth of the Christian faith, has said something correct regarding morality, and that the public negative consequences of his claim are something about which he does not have to care—even if it generally works the opposite of how it did. In general, as I mentioned, it is the truths that the Church proposes that are a stone of scandal for the world and that are persecuted. This is the clear evangelical message. When a Pope says, for example, that divorce, adultery, euthanasia, contraception, or homosexual acts are not acts of love, he must not worry about the scandal of the world in the face of such claims because he is no greater than his Master.

However, the principle works the same way in both senses. Whether the world tears its clothes in the face of the Pope's statements or welcomes them with open arms, he must not worry too much about any false and instrumental uses of them or of hypothetical international riots caused by them. If he affirms certain truths of Catholic morality, he can testify to them in good conscience to the world without caring for anything other than his duty to testify to them, even if such testimony is uncomfortable or unwelcome to some. We must therefore ask ourselves whether the idea that "vaccination is an act of love" can fall into this category of truth because, if it does, then one should in no way criticize the Pope for having proclaimed it. Indeed, he should be praised for the courage to testify to an inconvenient truth of faith at a time when it is urgent to do so. There is no way out, then; we must necessarily enter into the merits of the question.

1.1. Is it True that Getting Vaccinated Is an Act of Love? Moral Conscience and Common Sense

To answer this question, it is necessary to return to the foundations of moral choice starting first from common sense, because authentic morality cannot be in total contradiction with common sense. It can sometimes be difficult to understand, but never incomprehensible, and certainly in line with the *sensus fidei*: that is, with the supernatural understanding of the faith that the people of God, who are the Mystical Body of Christ and are assisted by the Spirit of Truth, have in history.[12]

12 Second Vatican Ecumenical Council, Dogmatic Constitution on the Church *Lumen Gentium*, n. 12: "The holy people of God shares also in Christ's prophetic office; it spreads abroad a living witness to Him, especially by means of a life of faith and charity and by offering to God a sacrifice of praise, the tribute of lips which give praise to His name (Heb. 13:15). The entire body of the faithful, anointed as they are by the Holy One (Jn. 2:20, 27), cannot err in matters of belief. They manifest this special property by means of the whole peoples' supernatural discernment in matters of faith when "from the Bishops down to the last of the lay faithful" [S. Augustine, *De Praed. Sanct.* 14,27: PL 44, 980] they show universal agreement in matters of faith and morals. That discernment in matters of faith is aroused and sustained by the Spirit of truth. It is exercised under the guidance of the sacred teaching authority, in faithful and respectful obedience to which the people of God accepts that which is not just the word of men but truly the word of God (1 Thess. 2:13). Through it, the people of God adheres unwaveringly to the faith given once and for all to the saints (Jud. 3), penetrates it more deeply with right thinking, and applies it more fully in its life."

I personally know many people who have had and have reasonable doubts about vaccines, not in general but with respect to specific cases. I also know many who got vaccinated and who really didn't care about others. They got vaccinated in order to return to a more comfortable life or to their usual selfish life. From this point of view, it is already reasonable to deduce that both choices, to get vaccinated or not to get vaccinated, can potentially be qualified as acts of love based on the circumstances and the intentionality of those who carry them out. Certainly, it cannot be said *a priori* that those who decide not to get vaccinated, or not to have a person who depends on them be vaccinated, do not do so as a choice of love. Moral judgment obviously presupposes some more data.

Imagine someone who knows the meaning of the emergency or conditional authorization of anti-Covid vaccines, who also knows the changing risk-benefit ratios of vaccines based on age and personal health conditions, who is aware of the changing risk assessment of the contagion on the basis of one's personal conditions (which, for example, allow one to live with one's family in reasonable isolation), who knows that neither his nor his family members have Covid and that therefore they are not contagious or dangerous to others, and who also realizes that the human person is the principal common good of the family and of the political community and that, therefore, moral duty towards oneself and one's loved ones coincides with moral duty towards the best good of the political community.

Imagine that this person, after reflecting a lot on the issue and taking note of the discordant opinions present among the experts, the discordant data in the various states, as well as the different political measures adopted in the various countries of the world, decides that it is prudent to have his grandfather vaccinated, but not a child of his own. Given the doubt that characterizes human choices, this person also prays a lot that he is doing the right thing. How could one say of such a person's choice that it is not an act of love? How could it be said that this choice does not respect the common good? Saying this would deny any value to moral conscience, making a person of good conscience pass for a bad person. Would it make sense to try to impose on this person the obligation (moral or legal) to have his child vaccinated by fully replacing his prudent reasoning about what is more appropriate for his child in the light of all the relevant circumstances and factors? Wouldn't such an attempt deny, even by common sense, the very foundations of Catholic moral doctrine?

1.2. Conscience as the Proximate Norm of Ethical Choice

Let's focus more fully now on moral conscience and on why it is so important for ethics and for the Christian. In classical and Christian morality, moral conscience plays a fundamental role because it is the proximate rule of moral action; it is the meeting point between the law of God and concrete action; it is the norm that decides the goodness or badness of a human being. In the words of St. John Paul II, moral conscience is "the place, the sacred place where God speaks to man."[13]

> "According to Saint Paul, conscience in a certain sense confronts man with the law, and thus becomes a *"witness" for man:* a witness of his own faithfulness or unfaithfulness with regard to the law, of his essential moral rectitude or iniquity. Conscience is the *only* witness, since what takes place in the heart of the person is hidden from the eyes of everyone outside. Conscience makes its witness known only to the person himself. And, in turn, only the person himself knows what his own response is to the voice of conscience."[14]

---

13 See John Paul II, Encyclical Letter *Veritatis Splendor* (VS), 6 August 1993, n. 58.

14 Ibid. n. 57.

Moral conscience is one of the most sublime points in which Christian morality elevates classical morality, recognizing together the objectivity of the moral law, the radical freedom and responsibility of the human being, and the ultimate criterion of his responsibility. The moral law is objective but must be applied in the here and in now of the extremely complex life that we live every day.[15] This application is like a very difficult sentence written by a careful magistrate. The sentence does not eliminate the laws but makes them live in the reality of the concrete case. Without the judgment of conscience (or without the sentence), there would be no moral life, and the law could not be applied.

> "Whereas the natural law discloses the objective and universal demands of the moral good, conscience is the application of the law to a particular case; this application of the law thus becomes an inner dictate for the individual, a summons to do what is good in this particular situation. Conscience thus formulates *moral obligation* in the light of the natural law: it is the obligation to do what the individual, through the workings of his conscience, *knows* to be a good he is called to do *here and now.* The universality of the law and its obligation are acknowledged, not suppressed, once reason has established the law's application in concrete present circumstances. The judgment of conscience states "in an ultimate way" whether a certain particular kind of behaviour is in conformity with the law; it formulates the proximate norm of the morality of a voluntary act, "applying the objective law to a particular case [...]"

15 There is an almost perfect epistemological correspondence between the traditional Christian doctrine on moral conscience and the Aristotelian explanation of practical syllogism and *proairesis* or deliberate moral choice. I explain this correspondence in detail in my *From Aristotle to Thomas Aquinas: Natural Law, Practical Knowledge, and the Person* (St. Augustine's Press: South Bend, IN, 2021), ch. II.

> "Consequently *in the practical judgment of conscience,* which imposes on the person the obligation to perform a given act, *the link between freedom and truth is made manifest.*"[16]

Moral conscience is the measure and foundation of the responsibility of the human person and of his rights to freedom. At the end of life, we will be judged based on the judgments of our conscience, which at times we will have taken seriously and have followed, doing good, and which at times we will have neglected or ignored, doing evil. Even if, by hypothesis, we had done a good thing against conscience, we would not be exempt from responsibility precisely because the ultimate rule of our action is our conscience and not the conscience or opinion of someone else.

> "The truth about the moral good, stated in the law of reason, is recognized practically and concretely by the *prudent judgment* of conscience. We call that man prudent who chooses in conformity with this judgment.
>
> Conscience enables one to assume *responsibility* for the acts performed. If man commits evil, the just judgment of conscience can remain within him as the witness to the universal truth of the good, at the same time as the evil of his particular choice [....]
>
> Man has the right to act in conscience and in freedom so as personally to make moral decisions. "He must not be forced to act contrary to his conscience [....]
>
> A human being must always obey the certain judgment of his conscience."[17]

These references to the Christian doctrine on moral conscience bring us back to common sense and the profound respect that must be shown for people's moral choices. They bring us

16 VS, nn. 59-61.

17 Catechism of the Catholic Church (CCC), nn. 1780-82, 1790.

back to the duty to help form conscience, not to impose hypothetical solutions to concrete cases from the outside. The Church has always been a teacher of respect for moral conscience, even in confessions, which are based on listening to penitents and not on investigative inquiries into what they tell the priest. With respect to moral conscience, one's duty is to help others to gather all the information necessary to make the best ethical choice, including, in the case of anti-Covid vaccines, risk-benefit assessments with respect to age or one's family and individual medical histories. Telling the doubtful conscience of the individual to get vaccinated "and that's that" is profoundly wrong and unfair already even according to common sense, without even applying the thousand-year old doctrine on moral conscience.

Let me emphasize this again due to its importance. The formation of a moral conscience involves exposure to the truth about the question on which it will have to decide. The more correct information you have, the better your choice will be. Trying to convince someone by giving them certainties that are not there is morally wrong. Trying to hide relevant information to get a person to act in a certain way is morally wrong. Trying to manipulate the truth or available information in a way that makes people choose in a certain way is highly immoral. Perhaps the main problem of moral conscience with respect to the choice of anti-Covid vaccines, as we will see, is the highly ambiguous, ideological, and manipulative context that has affected and corrupted the media and political authorities.

1.3. Reasoning and Sources of Morality

But how does conscience work? How does the agent, the ethical subject, apply moral law to a concrete case? Here, too, classical morality and Catholic doctrine are very clear. Moral conscience is about reasoning:

> "Saint Paul does not merely acknowledge that conscience acts as a "witness"; he also reveals the way in which conscience

performs that function. He speaks of "conflicting thoughts" which accuse or excuse the Gentiles with regard to their behaviour (cf. *Rom* 2:15). The term "conflicting thoughts" clarifies the precise nature of conscience: it is a *moral judgment about man and his actions,* a judgment either of acquittal or of condemnation, according as human acts are in conformity or not with the law of God written on the heart. In the same text the Apostle clearly speaks of the judgment of actions, the judgment of their author and the moment when that judgment will be definitively rendered: "(This will take place) on that day when, according to my Gospel, God judges the secrets of men by Christ Jesus" (*Rom* 2:16)."[18]

"*Conscience is a judgment of reason by which the human person recognizes the moral quality of a concrete act.*"[19]

Moral conscience is therefore a person's reasoning on the moral quality of a concrete act. And how is the moral quality of this act assessed? On this point, following the tradition of Aristotelian moral philosophy as taken up by scholasticism and, in particular, by St. Thomas Aquinas, the Catholic Church has developed, even at the catechetical level, the so-called doctrine according to which the morality of human acts depends on three elements. In these words from the Catechism,

"The morality of human acts depends on: the object chosen; the end in view or the intention; the circumstances of the action."

"A *morally good* act requires the goodness of the object, of the end, and of the circumstances together. "[20]

Therefore, to perform a good act, or an act of love, one must be certain in conscience that one is doing the objectively

18 VS, n. 59.

19 CCC, n. 1796.

20 CCC, nn. 1750, 1755.

right thing, in the right circumstances, and also that one is doing so with the right intention for its end. This clarification alone is also sufficient to conclude that it is impossible to say per se that getting vaccinated is an act of love. Even an act as pure as giving a kiss to one's mother, if done in the wrong circumstances and with the wrong intention, could be a morally bad act; and even an objectively bad act, such as slapping someone, if done in the right circumstances and with the right intention, could be a morally good act. This is not subjectivism, of course, it is understanding that the objectivity of the ethical choice depends on a plurality of elements, including intentional ones.

This book is arranged, even from a systematic point of view, on the study of the moral choice of using or not using anti-Covid vaccines through the specific analysis of object, circumstances, and end. The preponderant part concerns the circumstances, to which most of the chapters are dedicated, also because, for reasons that I will clarify, analysis of the circumstances partially comprehends analysis of the object. Both the general explanation of the end and the analysis of the relevant ends will be made in the last part, after the analysis of the circumstances. This is more correct both methodologically and systematically, and it also facilitates the understanding of the difference between the objective morality of the act and the subjective morality of the act: that is, that which depends on the intention of the agent.

1.4. An Important Clarification on Harm, on the Whole, and on the Part

It may seem strange to some to define 'slapping' as an objectively evil act. Among other things, haven't I just said that the goodness or badness of an act depends on a plurality of elements? How can I call it evil before evaluating all elements? The answer to this question is simple: the evaluation of the moral act presupposes, as I said, the evaluation of the goodness or badness of each single element of the act. In this case, it is therefore necessary to understand whether 'slapping' is bad from the point of view of the object, even before evaluating the end or the circumstances.[21]

From this point of view, therefore, consider that giving a slap objectively involves damage (whether slight or serious) to the body, and damage is always, as such, an evil. In classical and Christian morality, there is an objective hierarchy between goods, such that, for example, the goods of the spirit (such as freedom or faith) are superior to the goods of the body (such as health) and the goods of the body are superior to those of external goods (like properties).[22] If my eye causes me to sin, it is better for me to pluck it out and throw it away (Mark 9:47). If my child is sick and in need of expensive care, it is best for me to sell my car and forgo my vacation.

Evil, or damage to a lower good, can only be justified by the pursuit of a higher good and, ultimately, of the ultimate end. Irreparable damage to an inferior good can only be justified by a relationship of necessity with respect to the pursuit of a superior good (one can, for example, amputate a leg if doing so is a neces-

---

21 Intrinsically evil acts, that is, those whose wickedness, by hypothesis, depends solely on the object, are called this, adding the qualification 'intrinsically,' precisely to distinguish them from the mere ethical evaluation of the object as a single element of the act.

22 As I have already said, this work is not a scientific essay on fundamental ethical theory. It is a scientific essay on applied ethics that can be read by everyone regardless of the most fundamental critical issues of philosophy. I cannot therefore go into too much detail on sophisticated concepts of ethics and theory of action. For a more technical explanation of the hierarchy of goods involved in moral choice (and with particular attention to the thought of the doctor par excellence of the Catholic Church, St. Thomas Aquinas), I refer to the third chapter of my book, *God and the Natural Law* (St. Augustine's Press, South Bend, IN, 2002). Moreover, for further information on the moral good, the person, ethical choice, and the political good, see my *From Aristotle to Thomas Aquinas: Natural Law, Practical Knowledge, and the Person*, cit.

sary condition to save the patient). This does not imply that evil can be done for some future good to come, because the good of the part is functional to the good of the whole; therefore, it is inherent in the nature of the part that it can be sacrificed for the good of the whole. When the whole is in danger, the good of the part is to be sacrificed if needed in order to save the whole. The entire penal system is based on this principle. Punishment is bad by definition. If it were not, it would lose its very reason for existing. However, it is an evil that is justified with respect to the circumstances and the higher end to which it is ordered.

One can never sacrifice, however, an essential part of the whole, such as the brain with respect to the body or the innocent person with respect to the political community. This is the basic reason why utilitarianism as a political theory is wrong: because the innocent person is an essential and constitutive part of the political community. A state that sacrificed an innocent would deny itself, destroy its brain, and deny its ultimate end.[23] I will have to return to this point because, in times of crisis, utilitarianism is the easiest and most insidious temptation for both the individual and the community. When people are afraid, they become selfish and utilitarian, especially if they are rich and wealthy: that is, if they have so much to lose, like the rich young man in the Gospel, who sadly turns away from Jesus. Utilitarianism prevailed with the atomic bomb in World War II and is prevailing even now, in many ways, with the anti-Covid vaccines.

23 I talk about this in my *Ritorno al diritto. Miti e leggende della scienza giuridica moderna*, II edition (Phronesis Editore: Palermo, 2018).

Chapter 2

The Moral Object and Vaccine

In the tradition of Western thought, starting, at least, from Aristotle, only so-called intrinsically evil acts (or moral absolutes) have been considered such as to be able to be ethically characterized by virtue of the object alone, putting aside circumstances and intention. For the Catholic Church, for example, it is a firm principle that

> "There are acts which, in and of themselves, independently of circumstances and intentions, are always gravely illicit by reason of their object."[24]

These acts (even for those who consider them such) are very few and, for the Catholic Church, are strictly within the responsibility of the magisterium (abortion, euthanasia, killing of the innocent, adultery, contraception, homosexual acts, etc.).

The most important thing we need to emphasize here is that intrinsically evil acts are all negative, and it could not be otherwise. In ethics, it is conceptually possible to say that something cannot be done whatever the end and the circumstances, but it is not possible to say absolutely that a certain thing must always be done whatever the circumstances and the end. On the positive side, for example, I can say that we must always love God, but that tells me nothing about the fact that now I might need to

24 CCC, n. 1756.

love God by eating a steak rather than by taking the children to the beach. I can say that if your child is in danger, you ought to save him, but this does not tell me anything about the concrete action you might take or ought to take now to try to save him, nor if, given the circumstances, it is actually possible to save him. "Truth be told" is a general valid precept; however, right now, instead of telling any truth, it might be better to eat ice cream or to shut up. The ethical choice is in the here and now, and all the potentialities of an individual's life cannot be exhausted in the abstract. Epistemologically, it is necessary to be able to distinguish between the truth value of the general rules and principles of action and that of specific indications on the here and now of an ethical choice.

> "In the case of the positive moral precepts, prudence always has the task of verifying that they apply in a specific situation, for example, in view of other duties which may be more important or urgent. But the negative moral precepts, those prohibiting certain concrete actions or kinds of behaviour as intrinsically evil, do not allow for any legitimate exception. They do not leave room, in any morally acceptable way, for the 'creativity' of any contrary determination whatsoever. Once the moral species of an action prohibited by a universal rule is concretely recognized, the only morally good act is that of obeying the moral law and of refraining from the action which it forbids."[25]

Let's also assume that a certain object, in the abstract, is always good compared to a certain good end, such as eating and sleeping or taking a certain drug are respectively good for staying healthy, living, and for treating or avoiding a disease. In these cases, I could say that, *in the abstract*, choosing this object for oneself or for others who depend on us, is an act of love towards oneself, towards others, and towards the common good (which is

25 VS, n. 67.

constituted above all by people). Yet I should clarify that this is an improper way (*secundum quid*) of speaking about the moral act, because in the concrete realm of the ethical choice (*simpliciter*), the act of love cannot depend on the mere material choice of that object.

Let's assume, for example, that we are the Pope and that we feel in conscience the moral duty to demonstrate in times of epidemic that God is Lord of the events of the world and that, therefore, we decide not to close Lourdes, and we go there on pilgrimage without vaccinating ourselves; or we decide to lead a procession with some relics of saints to ask God to stop the epidemic and we, to show the power of faith with facts, decide to lead the procession without vaccinating ourselves or covering our face with a mask. In a case like this, not getting vaccinated would be part of a higher act of love and faith, both because the good of faith is superior to the good of bodily life and because the power of God is superior to that of any virus.

Let's continue this thought experiment, and assume now that we, as the Pope, while believing that it would be good to get vaccinated, to give an example to our sheep, and trusting in God, decide not to do so until everyone else, up to the last of the faithful in the world, has been vaccinated. Even in this case, not getting vaccinated would undoubtedly be part of an act of superior love which would also demonstrate the primacy of faith, charity, and the power of God. Let's assume again that we are the Pope, but that now we are among the first people in the world to get vaccinated. We could have done it to give an example to everyone about a behavior that we believe everyone should imitate, or we could have done it simply out of fear of contagion, taking advantage of our privileged position at a time when very few in the world had access to the vaccine. In this case, the very material act of getting vaccinated among the first in the world could be either an act of love or an act of cowardice and selfishness.

This simple observation on the distinction between positive and negative precepts, coupled with the evident fact that the vaccine does not fall under any negative precept, is also sufficient in and of itself to clarify that getting vaccinated or not getting vaccinated cannot by itself, regardless of the circumstances and the end of the concrete action, be defined as a choice of love or hatred. Still, of course, there are many other factors to take into consideration.

2.1. The "Vaccine" as an Ambiguous Object

So far, I have assumed that getting vaccinated (against Covid) is an object of choice that in the abstract is always good for the purpose of health, but, by doing so, I am making some erroneous generalizations. In fact, the word "vaccine" is not a univocal term because there are many types of vaccines. Vaccines must be defined on the basis, at least, of the type of disease they tend to eradicate, the type of effectiveness they have, their side effects, the subjects or groups who may not be able to receive them, the risks depending on the compounds and techniques used to make them, the degree of experimentation involved in their production, the critical moral issues involved (for example, for the use, in producing them, of parts of aborted children), etc. This level of objective ambiguity of the term "vaccine" is enough for us to reject the idea that it could univocally identify, in the abstract, the moral object of a specific ethical choice.

The use of what anti-Covid vaccine would be an act of love? All? Always? Whatever the ethical critical issues and whatever the percentages of efficacy, risk, etc.? It would be enough to focus on just the one ethical issue that I have just mentioned to understand that the Pope's generalist statement was specifically contradicted by the Congregation for the Doctrine of the Faith itself when it stated that "*vaccines that have used cell lines from aborted fetuses in their research and production process*" cannot be used when there is the possibility of using others. In other words, according to the Congregation for the Doctrine of the Faith, the use of a vaccine is not always an act of love but could, on the contrary, be sinful based on the circumstances of the alternatives available.[26]

One wonders why the Pope has not bothered to underline this important exception, given that most of the faithful in the world have not even realized the existence of this ethical problem linked to the use of certain vaccines. It goes without saying, in any case, that if it is possible to differentiate between anti-Covid vaccines based on moral issues, it must also be so with respect to any other relevant factor. Pastors should therefore help the faithful to make the most appropriate ethical choices by informing them in the best possible way rather than trying to direct them ambiguously towards a hypothetical generalizing solution valid for all and in all cases.

Even if we wanted to better qualify the "vaccine" object by saying, for example, that "vaccinating with Pfizer[27] against Covid is an act of love," there would remain the problem of clarifying whether the object "Pfizer vaccine against Covid" is the same ethical object in the cases, for example, of the moral choices of a ninety-year-old without pathologies, of a person who has recovered from Covid, of a two-year-old child, or of a family living in the countryside. In other words, it can be argued that the "Pfizer vaccine against Covid" as a tool (even before considering the cir-

---

26 See Congregation for the Doctrine of the Faith, "Note on the morality of using some anti-Covid-19 vaccines," December 21, 2020, URL: https://press.vatican.va/content/salastampa/it/bollettino/pubblico/2020/12/21/0681/01591.html. Frankly, I am very sorry to read documents of the Church in which, probably out of respect for the world, they do not use the term "child," but the hideous and depersonalizing "fetus," which is a term promoted *ad hoc* to favor abortion culture. Furthermore, I do not intend here to endorse the ethical reasoning present in the aforementioned note, but only to highlight the contrast between it and the Pope's generalizing statement on vaccination as an act of love.
27 Because, allegedly, it provides more protection than AstraZeneca or other Covid vaccines.

cumstances as an element of analysis other than the object) should not be characterized, from an objective point of view, with regard to an end which may be different for different subjects, and which would therefore make it, for these subjects, an *objectively different instrument.*

2.1.1. Object and End

Here it is easy to get confused between object, end, and circumstances. It is crucial to understand that these terms are analogical and that the precise scope of their predication must always be understood correctly. An object, or a tool, is always defined based on its purpose or function. The hammer cannot be objectively defined irrespective of the purpose of driving the nails. When I rationally choose to use the hammer as a hammer, therefore, I make that end mine even with respect to the intentionality of my actions. It is my action that makes the hammer a hammer.

The objective end of the hammer tool will therefore enter the intentional description of my action or ethical choice, which still can also respond to a further purpose. I use the hammer to drive some nails to build a Nativity stable with my son. Here my action has at least one ultimate end that could be described as the love of God that leads me to build the stable; a penultimate goal, if you like, which is the love of my son that leads me to do something with him while teaching him to love God (by building the stable together); and a near or immediate end that coincides with driving nails using the hammer.

The analysis of moral action based on the agent's ends does not exclude the analysis of the object of the act with respect to its function, which requires an understanding of what makes that object objectively suitable for its purpose or function. A typical mistake made in ethics is not to understand that the evaluation of the object of the action implies in itself the understanding of an end which, with respect to the object, has a defining character, and that, when the agent decides to use that object, by default enters the ethical intentionality of the agent himself.

Whatever the ulterior end that the agent intends, his moral intentionality will also include the acceptance and use of the end of the chosen object. I repeat, it is the agent who makes the hammer a hammer.

The case is different when the agent uses the hammer not as a hammer, for example by slipping it under a wardrobe that risks falling due to a broken leg, or by placing it on sheets of paper to prevent the wind from carrying them away. In these cases, the intentional action does not make the objective end of the hammer its own because the objective being of the hammer is only accidental compared to the action that is being performed. For both of those actions, a stone, or a piece of marble, or a thousand other things could have been used, precisely because they are not actions for which you need a hammer. The action, therefore, in this case, does not make the hammer a hammer; on the contrary, it makes it something else: the leg of a wardrobe or a paperweight.

Let me give you a slightly more sophisticated ethical example, to be clearer. Contraception is, for the Catholic Church, an intrinsically evil action. However, using a contraceptive for therapeutic purposes or to defend against sexual violence could be morally lawful even for the Catholic Church. Saying this does not imply creating an exception to the intrinsically evil act, because there can be no exceptions to an act that is evil based on the object and regardless of any circumstance and end. So how is the absolute ban on choosing the "contraceptive" object reconciled with the apparent exception of using a contraceptive lawfully? It is reconciled precisely because the object of the act is defined according to an end to which it is structurally ordered: in the case of contraception, having sex while avoiding the risk of pregnancy; in the case of theft, appropriating someone else's property. If the same material instrument is used for completely different purposes, being a multifunctional instrument, then when it is used for therapeutic purposes or for defense, it is equivalent to a different ethical object. The contraceptive used for the purpose of wanting to enjoy "safe sex" is an objectively different tool from the one used to defend oneself (albeit, unfortunately, only partially) from violence. Here there is an objective difference similar to that of the hammer being used to keep the wardrobe from falling or to weigh down the papers.[28]

2.1.2. Object and Circumstances

A similar argument applies to the circumstances of the moral act. The identification of the object of human action necessarily implies some circumstances which, precisely because they define the object, are different from those that could be added to the evaluation of the action. Let's think back to the hammer. We have seen that the definition implies an intrinsic end. Let us now consider that the definition also implies some structural circumstances, especially those of a metal extremity (a head made of heavy and hard material) attached to a handle capable of conveying the multiplied action of a lever to the extremity. These elements, in a certain sense, are circumstances, but, in another sense, with respect to the instrument as such, they are not: they are part of its very definition.

When we ask ourselves about the object and circumstances of a moral act, we must understand that some circumstances are only apparently such because in reality they fall within the objective structure of the act itself. Some objects are not chosen, not because the circumstances are unfavorable, but because they are not the right objects.

A villa's limestone brick is objectively not good for the walls of a skyscraper, not because the circumstances of the skyscraper advise against it, but because some bricks are not made to support the walls of a skyscraper. It is not a matter of circumstances. Some bricks are not a suitable object of choice with respect to the purpose of building the walls of a skyscraper. The

28 For a more detailed analysis of this type of example related to sexual ethics, see my *From Aristotle to Thomas Aquinas*, cit.

tool is objectively defined based on the specific purpose to which it is ordered, and the specific purpose (skyscraper/villa, two-year-old child/80-year-old senior) could change the objective defining nature of the tool.[29]

Again, it is not the circumstances that change in these cases; it is the object of the moral act that also depends on some circumstances. The moral act is objectively defined according to the use of an instrument that has an intrinsic end and some intrinsic circumstances, but then it goes way beyond that instrument, towards other ends and other circumstances. The brick is not as such the object of a moral act, but building a house and living in it with one's family are. Like the bricks, the "Pfizer Covid vaccine" could be a different moral object in the case of an elderly person, a Covid survivor, or a child, because each of them could do something objectively different with it, and on the basis of different moral evaluations. I will return to these things in detail by talking about the specific circumstances of the different vaccines.

All this should not be a surprise precisely, because in ethics, from a technical point of view, there are circumstances that fall within the definition of the object and other circumstances that do not. Even the end, in absolute terms, is equivalent to a circumstance because, compared to a technical object that I happen to have in front of me, the fact of using it to drive a nail, to weigh down sheets of paper, or to support the weight of the wardrobe is, after all, a circumstance of my choice. I will not tire of repeating this. Both the term "circumstance" and the term "ob-

29 Of course, regarding the example of the limestone bricks and the skyscraper, I defer to the judgment of the engineers. Since this is not my professional field, it is enough that my example have sufficient analog value to clarify the ethical concept, but it does not need to have truth accuracy in the field of engineering and construction science. I sincerely hope that no one relies on this book to design a skyscraper or a villa in the countryside.

ject" and the term "end" are analogical, and one must always understand the specific semantic area of each usage we make of them. Each element of the action must be analogically characterized as an end, a circumstance, or as part of the object based on the context of the discourse and the individual moral act to which it refers.

Regarding the circumstances, we must always ask ourselves whether, in some cases, they are only apparently such because they fall instead within the definition of the object. Let's explore a final example to clarify this important aspect of moral and legal theory even better.

The belonging of an asset to others is a circumstance that falls within the definition of the moral object "theft" and therefore, with respect to theft, it is not a circumstance. In other words, in the absence of this "circumstance," there is no lesser theft; there is simply no theft at all (as in the absence of the handle that allows for leverage, you do not have the hammer). We can play analogically with words as much as we want but, in the end, we have to understand each other concerning the action and its object. The belonging of the goods to others does not even fall within the structural end of the object "theft" because whoever steals does not do it to take something away from others but to appropriate that something. If the thief enjoys taking something away from someone else, he commits an immoral act beyond that of the theft, whose specific structural intention is not to take it away from others, but to appropriate it for himself. The thief wants money; if he finds it on the street, he doesn't have to bother taking it from someone. Taking property away from others is a defining circumstance of the "theft" object, different from the intentional defining circumstance of the same object.

Some characteristics of the vaccine related to its use on different subjects could take on an objective and not merely circumstantial definitional value. If the administration of a certain vaccine to a minor, for example, had the sole effect or advantage of protecting the elderly from infections transmitted by the minor, while the administration of that same vaccine to the elderly had the effect of protecting the latter from Covid, then that vaccine would be an objectively different tool, respectively, for minors and for the elderly, as the hammer is different from the paperweight. Even if we limit ourselves to the only objective definition of the "vaccine" tool, therefore, there are too many variables at stake to be able to make statements, in generalizing and absolute terms, about its objective ethical goodness. The very idea of wanting to do so, to use an expression of Thomas Aquinas, *risibile videtur*.

2.2. The Vaccine as an Instrumental Moral Object

In the previous section, I hypothesized that the vaccine is an abstractly good object with respect to the end of health, but I raised the doubt that it may not be possible to define it in an objectively univocal way without considering the specific type (Pfizer, etc.) and the different way in which it is a *tool* with respect to different situations and people. Now I need to be more precise by saying that the vaccine, even overcoming those definitional difficulties, remains a mere instrumental good with respect to a relative end, and it is therefore not radically possible to define it per se as good: that is, one cannot say that using it is per se an act of love.

In ethics, it is essential to distinguish between good or end in a relative sense and good or end in an absolute sense. The ethical choice is good when it responds to the absolute good of the person and not only to a relative good such as, for example, health. The case of medicine is, in fact, often used as a typical example to explain this difference, and I myself have done it several times.[30] If a physician (or a virologist, biologist, epidemiologist)

30 See, e.g., R. Spaemann, *Basic Moral Concepts*, trans. T. J. Armstrong (London and New York: Routledge, 1989), pp. 19-31, 87-99; F. Di

(continued on the next page)

tells me that "I *ought* to take a certain drug," he makes a statement that has a scientific significance only with respect to his discipline. In fact, he could tell me that, according to his professional health competence, that drug is what, in my state of health, I have to use. However, a human being is not just health, and moral duty is all-encompassing. The doctor has no competence to tell me whether taking that drug corresponds to my ultimate good as a person and whether it will let me go to heaven (to put it in eschatological terms).

The physician may tell me I need to stay in bed, but my highest duty right now may require getting up and going to help my child. The relative duty of medical judgment is not the absolute duty of moral choice. Moral duty is an evaluation, not of the relative good of medicine (with respect to health), but of the absolute good with respect to the ultimate end of the person (which includes, for example, duties towards the family, towards the entire human community and towards God). A person, for example, could believe that, in the current context, not getting vaccinated, despite the risks of Covid, is his moral duty, for the following reasons (among other things): a) to demonstrate to the state that it is wrong to try to subjugate all citizens to a single authoritarian thought and b) to tell the church that it is placing dubious health policies before faith in God and revealed truth, with the consequence of alienating many people from the true faith, thereby creating serious and useless divisions within the people of God. To such an ethical reflection, right or wrong though it may be, the physician (or vir-*ologist*, and the entire group of *-ologists* parading on TV at the moment) as such could not object to anything because the good on which he is an expert is the relative good of health, not the absolute one of the ultimate end, or the ultimate salvation of the person and the world.

Blasi, *God and the Natural Law*, section 2.3.3. "The Formal Object of Ethics."

This is a distinction that judges know very well with respect to the opinions of the experts called to give relevant technical judgments during a court trial. Whatever the experts say (since generally they are more than one according to the number of parties in the trial), the judge must take into account all the relevant factors in the process and the rules of law. The expert may well be right, but he may express in a technical way only one of the relevant elements of a certain court case. Formally, there is always a difference between the expert opinion (of the technician) and the verdict (of the judge). Unfortunately, however, this simple distinction is not clear to many individual moral subjects and to many politicians when they think that their choices must be entirely determined by a certain technical opinion (provided it exists and is univocal). A moral choice, both individual and political, must look at the entire universe of the person and the community, which cannot be superseded by any technical opinion as such. The technical opinion is to the ethical choice as one of the factors is to the whole, and the technician must always distinguish his specialist opinion from his moral and political opinions (which have the same value as anyone else's).

Even under the more technical aspect that I have just addressed, concerning the nature of the "vaccine" as a medical tool (relative good) and as a potential object of moral choice (absolute good), to say that getting vaccinated is an act of love appears to represent a reversal of ethics (or of the absolute good) with respect to medicine (relative good): a reversal that is equivalent to an unacceptable enslavement of ethics to medicine and of the goods of the spirit to those of the body. Health can never and under no circumstance rise to become the ultimate criterion for evaluating the moral good.

Some objectors tell the many believers who have doubts about the vaccines that God wants human beings to live, meaning that, in this moment of crisis, health must be put first and one ought to get vaccinated for the good of all. There are undue generalizations involved in this type of objection, which this book intends to address and clarify. Furthermore, for Christians, ethical evaluation always reveals God's will, which should be carefully examined in light of the entire revealed truth. Aside from more specific answers and arguments that I will develop later, however, here I would like to interrupt my purely philosophical (and not theological) reasoning for a moment to react to this objection as I think a believer should instinctively react.

God wants us to live, of course, but He has also created a world in which one dies, and ultimately He wants human beings to earn eternal life in the afterlife with a faith capable of going beyond the good of the body. Sacred history is a history in which one dies for God and in which faith is true when it looks beyond the present life. Abraham is the hero of faith because he did not hesitate to sacrifice his only son (who was also a political asset, as Abraham's only descendant). The passage from the Bible on Abraham is very difficult to interpret, but not because of the aspect that makes Abraham the hero of faith. The ultimate destiny of man is not in this world, and for this reason the ultimate criterion of moral good cannot be health. The believer cannot, by his own DNA, submit all the other criteria of choice, including the mystery of God's will and the otherworldly destiny of human existence, to the mere pursuit of physical health.

The theological digression is over. Let's return to philosophy and, from this point onward, as promised in the Introduction, there will be no further references to specific conceptual approaches focused on the Catholic or Christian tradition in this book.

Chapter 3

The Vaccines and the Circumstances of the Moral Act

We now move from our discourse on the object to that on circumstances, that is, to the second of the three elements with which conscience must evaluate the moral quality of the human act. Given the uncertainty of the objective definition of the "anti-Covid vaccine" tool, it will be good to approach the circumstances regardless of the assessment of whether or not some of them can be considered as defining the object. This, in fact, is a very interesting theoretical question, but also of little use in relation to the objectives of this text, which, as I said in the introduction, do not concern fundamental theory but applied ethics.

In this chapter, I will not yet address the heart of the individual circumstances relating to the ethical choice of the anti-Covid vaccine. The identification and analysis of individual circumstances comprises a large part of the entire book and are a theme that will be explored in subsequent chapters. It is also an open-ended discourse, which in itself cannot be exhausted, just as the life and existence of people as moral agents cannot be exhausted in the abstract. This is still an architectural framing chapter of the question in which, having already clarified the conceptual terms of the object of the moral act, I will have to introduce, in general, the most important conceptual distinctions relating to the circumstances of the moral act that surround the possible choice of anti-Covid vaccines.

3.1. Number, Identification, and Relevance of the Circumstances

We must keep in mind, as I have already said, that the circumstances of the moral act are not limited in number, and that part of the work of the ethical subject (both individual and political) is precisely that of trying to identify them and to weigh them for the purposes of moral choice. If this book were intended to be exhaustive, it would start from a flawed logical and methodological premise and would therefore be doomed to failure.

The work of the ethics expert, concerning both the circumstances and the ends, is initially made complicated by the methodological need to move with great attention and discernment between objective and subjective plans.

3.1.1. Internal Point of View

Ethics lies above all in the point of view of the person who acts, because it concerns freedom and what makes us good or bad by doing what we choose to do. Ethics cannot be imposed from the outside. For this reason, radical freedom of conscience is what no slavery or totalitarianism can ever take away from a person. You can put a person in prison, you can tie him up and torture him, you can even kill him, but you can never take away his freedom to be what he chooses to be, until the end. Ethics was born with Socrates when this giant of thought realized that the human being rises inwardly above any power of nature and finds in himself his own strength and his own ultimate fulfillment. Socrates' ethics teach us the primacy of self-control (*enkrateia*), autonomy (*autarkeia*), and the inner enjoyment of one's freedom (*eleutheria*), which are ultimately able to conquer any tyrant as well as the impulses of our own nature. Even before the external world, ethics has as its object the interior one. It has as its object the person, his virtues, and his vices.

Why this premise? Because when reflecting on the circumstances and the relevant purposes of the ethical choice, the expert must first ask himself what is important or relevant, in a certain area of action, for the person who moves or acts in that area. If there is a question that profoundly affects someone's choices, the ethics expert cannot disdain it or put it aside on the hypothetical assumption that it is not an objective or relevant issue. It is relevant because it affects the ethical choice. It is objective because it is relevant to whoever acts. How objective it really is and how relevant it must be is what the expert must try to understand and argue at a later time. The expert must learn to switch points of view. The third point of view of the observing scholar must recognize that, from the internal point of view of the agent, a question could be seen and experienced as objective and relevant. In moral philosophy, a distinction is made, in this regard, between the point of view of the first person and that of the third person, or between the internal and external points of view.

In fundamental ethics, an endless chapter would open here on how one can ultimately distinguish between objective and subjective. What my wife thinks about certain matters is important to me. For a third party observer, this could be a subjective element with respect to choice. But if for husbands it is generally important what their wives think, is it still a subjective element or has it become objective? For marketers it is certainly objective because, often, the husband buys something just because his wife likes it. It would be stupid, or not objective from a marketing point of view, not to use this data. And if the husband does it, if he buys something, or buys one thing instead of something else, just because his wife likes it, does he act in an arbitrary way with respect to the objectivity of the product or it is rather an objective circumstance of his choice that, for him, under certain conditions, buying that product is indifferent compared to the importance of pleasing his wife? If, for a father, taking home food for his children is more important than health, it is useless to keep telling him that it is not objective to leave the house to go to work while still being sick. That health can be more important than children is a subjective and wrong medical point of view: it is bad medicine. And who decides whether a certain medical or health risk is objectively worse than another? Often, the difference between objective and subjective is a matter of points of view between which the ethics expert must learn to distinguish.

Let's turn to Covid. There are millions of people in the world who, right now, fear the attack on their freedom more than they fear the virus. The politician who thinks this is a subjective issue with respect to the pandemic only proves that he does not know how to step outside of his own point of view, and he will end up doing his job badly. It is objective that if (political or media) power insults and humiliates intelligence and freedom too much, the best citizens will finally stand up to react with the power of their word and example, while the mediocre citizens will often react violently by refusing, at that point, any rational discussion. From this point of view, those who think that their truth about anti-Covid vaccines legitimizes the current campaign of arrogant, insulting, and one-sided media and institutional hammering are underestimating two objective aspects of the question: the more energetic opposing reaction from the best citizens in the society, and the opposing reaction tending to violence from the worst. These are among the reasons why some good scholars who have been working on vaccines for many years have argued that the exaggerations on the subject of vaccines in the current management of the pandemic have ruined twenty or thirty years of constructive work done to encourage the use of vaccines and to make them more acceptable even to the reluctant.[31]

---

31 See, e.g., M. Kulldorff, Ph.D., professor of medicine at Harvard Medical School, biostatistician and epidemiologist at Brigham and Women's Hospital and former member of the scientific advisory committees of the FDA and the American CDC (*Centers for Disease Control and Prevention*), "Interview by J. Jekielek," *American Thought Leaders*, August 10, 2021, URL: https://www.theepochtimes.com/harvard-epidemiologist-martin-kulldorff-on-vaccine-passports-the-delta-variant-and-the-covid-public-

(continued on the next page)

Let's get back to us. When we try to identify the circumstances relevant to the moral choice, we must first make the matter personal, both for others and for ourselves. What are the elements that, in a certain context, potentially influence people's ethical choice? What are the ones that affect mine? What is important to me, as an ethical subject, for my decision-making? This second type of questioning does not insert a subjectivist element into moral reasoning. It makes it authentic and serves to facilitate the identification of relevant circumstances. In fact, if something that is not relevant to the scholar is instead relevant to all or most of the subjects involved, it is more likely that the ethics scholar has not understood or interpreted it well. If parents were generally indifferent to their children and vice versa, family ethics would simply not exist, and the scholar would have very little to say about it.

Asking ourselves what is relevant for us and for the other subjects involved is not decisive at the theoretical level, but it is very useful for heuristic purposes. Furthermore, the discovery or underlining of a relevant factor will normally arouse immediate interest or curiosity on the part of the moral agent and will eventually influence his choice. This is a great test for the scholar. Maybe a certain person had not thought about that particular circumstance and had been, up to that moment, indifferent to it only for this reason, that he did not know about it or had not contextualized it. Yet in hearing it now, clearly, in the context of moral action that is important to him, his eyes immediately light

---

health-fiasco_3942556.html?fbclid=IwAR0aVLloiP-pAi3jGyRBzV-zXXT18U9JN17J9w5PnAOLsRyzN5sGWPjPEEQ: "Those who are pushing these vaccine mandates and vaccine passports—vaccine fanatics, I would call them—to me they have done much more damage during this one year than the anti-vaxxers have done in two decades. I would even say that these vaccine fanatics, they are the biggest anti-vaxxers that we have right now. They're doing so much more damage to vaccine confidence than anybody else."

up and his attention is awakened. This is the sign that it was indeed a relevant circumstance that the scholar had to analyze and evaluate correctly.

3.1.2. External Point of View

The scholar cannot invent the importance of things. What is important to people is a starting point for him (to be understood and analyzed carefully, as I said), not a conclusion. But he can work on the truth because the human being is the only being whose own action, as Aristotle said, is the mysterious result, not of physical forces and instincts, but of *nous* and *logos*, intellect and reason. The reason why this is mysterious is that the intellect itself does not move anything, but this is one of those questions of fundamental ethics (extremely difficult at that) that goes far beyond the limits and meaning of this book.[32]

As I have already emphasized since the Introduction, moral choice (or rational action) is based both on the knowledge that the intellect has of what one does and on the will or freedom to do it. The intellect understands and reasons; the will desires and chooses. The two things act in full dialectic and synergy in the moral conscience. This is where the scholar can begin more constructive and objective work because the moral agent is not just an animal that desires but is an animal that thinks about what to do and is therefore able to understand and evaluate his own desires or inclinations in the light of the objective truth of the situation. The scholar, then, after having considered the agent's internal point of view, can also consider the external and objec-

---

32 On this point, let me refer to my *From Aristotle to Thomas Aquinas*, op. cit., esp., ch. II, "Practical Syllogism, *Proairesis*, and the Virtues: Toward a Reconciliation of Virtue Ethics and Natural Law Ethics," whose previous version had been published in *New Things & Old Things*, 1/2004, and is also available in Italian in my *Conoscenza pratica, teoria dell'azione e bene politico* (Rubbettino: Soveria Mannelli, 2006).

tive features of the area involved in the action, and bring the two things into synergy.

The human being is multifaceted. There are so many things that are important to him (health, family, freedom, truth, friendship, justice, professional fulfillment, God, etc.) and so many ways to observe each of them. Moral action, however, implies a hierarchy that allows you to choose in the here and now. Let's not be concerned about whether this hierarchy is ultimately to be understood as objective or subjective. This is another question of fundamental ethics that I am not interested in at the moment and about which I have written extensively (and in a much more boring way) elsewhere.[33]

We all generally agree that hierarchy is necessary, even among scholars. If I now stop writing this book for a while so that I can eat or change the baby's diaper, it means that there are criteria for my action (almost always implicit and spontaneous) that tell me what is most important to do in the different moments of my day and life. At such a moment, my little girl moves to first position in importance, so I stop writing. If there are no reasons that keep her in the first position of importance with respect to the book, I will be able to write it again later—otherwise the book can also go down the drain, because in my life, taking care of my daughter or my son or my wife are hierarchically more important things than writing the book. Without hierarchy, and with so many beautiful and important things to do in life, an agent could not move.

When the scholar adopts the external point of view, he can reflect and make others reflect on the different important human goods, on the way in which they interact, on the way in which sometimes or always one prevails over another, on the reasons

33 See, e.g., F. Di Blasi, *John Finnis* (Phronesis: Palermo, 2008); *God and the Natural Law*, cit.; "I Valori Fondamentali nella Teoria Neoclassica della Legge Naturale," *Rivista Internazionale di Filosofia del Diritto*, 2/1999.

why they are important, and/or on the reasons by which they can be pursued for better or worse.

Let's assume, for example, that for a Catholic, it is very important to obey what the Pope and the President of his state say, to the point of questioning oneself, compared to one's own doubts about vaccines, in listening to the pressures to get vaccinated by these authorities. The importance that Catholics attach to the Pope's or to the President's statements is an objective thing both internally and externally, but it relates respectively to the good of faith and the common good, and neither of these two goods implies that technical or ethical opinions on vaccines from the Pope and the President are better or more reliable than ours and those of many experts in the field. Paradoxically, in this specific case, the President's opinion could have greater ethical relevance than the Pope's, but I will have to return to these things later in a more analytical way. Here I just want to underline that a circumstance which is relevant and objective from someone's internal point of view ("the Pope said so," "the President said so")—and which is objective, at its level (faith, common good), even from an external point of view—can become irrelevant to the scrutiny of reason. In a case like this, the scholar who has understood the internal relevance of the circumstance without discarding it or ignoring it a priori, can really be of help when, as a third observer, he evaluates and explains its actual objective significance.

To summarize: when identifying or evaluating both the circumstances and the ends relevant to the ethical choice, one must first of all do so from the internal point of view, so as to be sure to keep in touch with reality, not to neglect anything important, and not to block a priori a constructive dialogue with the stakeholders, so to speak. Then, the study must also be undertaken from the external point of view of the third party observer, which generally originates from the most evident data available about the specific case regardless of the subjective points of view of the interested parties

3.2. Circumstances Internal and External to the Vaccine

Regarding the specific circumstances of the moral act concerning the vaccine, we must first distinguish between circumstances that we could call internal and circumstances that we could call external to the anti-Covid vaccine. It is evident, in fact, that there may be elements that influence the moral choice to get vaccinated or not to get vaccinated that have nothing to do with the intrinsic characteristics of the vaccine or have no direct bearing on it.

Think, for example, of trust, that is, the value we can or should give to the information that the authorities provide us. How much can and should the fact, for example, that the President of our state has advised us to get vaccinated or that the news or some experts give certain indications about this, affect our choice?

3.2.1. External Circumstances and Ends

Here, however, there is an ambiguity that must be avoided. Almost all the external circumstances that affect the choice to get vaccinated fall within the order of ends. That is, they concern the assessments of the good of health, seen as an end, with respect to different goods or ends that could lead the moral agent to get vaccinated or not to get vaccinated. Even the choice to get vaccinated in order to protect the people around us concerns our end, and it presupposes a previous evaluation of the object and the circumstances of the anti-Covid vaccine. In other words, if we have concluded that a certain vaccine is, here and now, the best tool to protect the people around us, and if this is our goal, then we will choose to be vaccinated with that vaccine. Otherwise, even based on the same evaluation of the object and the circumstances, we may decide not to get vaccinated.

Properly speaking, the ends are always external to the object and the circumstances and, therefore, when a circumstance is characterized as an end, it will be taken into consideration in the specific ethical treatment concerning ends. If there are reasons to address it immediately, it must be clarified that it is a circumstance linked to intentionality and not to the knowledge in itself of the act to be performed. I repeat that the difference between circumstances and ends is partly analogical and therefore we must not separate discourse about circumstances too far from that about ends. However, it is important to underline this because, in itself, the analysis of circumstances pertains to a merely cognitive phase of the action, while that of the ends to an intentional and appetitive-volitional phase. The ends are what attract our will and ultimately lead us to choose one way or the other.

The specific end involved in the choice of the vaccine is that of health (one's own or that of others). The ethical choice, however, as I have already clarified, is aimed at the absolute good of the person and not only at the person as (currently or only potentially) sick. Even in the case of ends, therefore, we could consider a theoretical distinction between internal ends, with respect to the choice of the vaccine, and external ends, which do not directly concern the good of health, but other goods of the person or his ultimate end.[34]

It goes without saying, as I like to always recall, that regarding external circumstances, regarding external goods or ends, and regarding the ultimate end, medical experts have no scientific competence; they can only speak of them in the same way as any other person of good conscience.

---

34 Again, I clarify to colleagues that I want to avoid unnecessary discussions of fundamental ethics. Consequently, I will never adopt in this book a limiting technical concept of ultimate end, but only the generic one of the deepest or most significant sense that can lead someone to make radical decisions that deny or sacrifice the other goods of the person. This is a contingent logical concept of ultimate end on which, in the context of this book and provisionally, a consensus can be generated and maintained.

With respect to external circumstances and ends, for example, the particular role of a subject could affect the intentionality of the ethical choice. Think of the examples given above in relation to the Pope, or even the case of a person with public responsibility who feels the need to demonstrate to his community the existence or importance of a superior ethical value. In this sense, depending on one's role or office, the choice not to get vaccinated could be comparable to that of going on a hunger strike. Objecting to those who go on hunger strike by stating that their action is contrary to the nutritional purpose of food would be ethically contradictory, because the act of striking presupposes that nutritional value, which is precisely being renounced to publicly demonstrate some hypothetically higher moral significance than health. It would also be ethically wrong to criticize those who are on a hunger strike by saying that they are not performing an act of love, or even that they are doing violence to society by forcing it to make certain decisions. From their point of view, in fact, they are performing an act of love higher than those who only care about physical health, and they are doing it precisely to ensure that society makes objectively better decisions for the common good.

Since the circumstances and ends external to the vaccine—and potentially relevant to each individual moral subject—not only cannot be exhausted in the abstract, as is the case for all circumstances and ends, but they are also much broader and more open to possibilities, even with respect to them it will not be possible to say, in absolute and abstract terms, whether the choice to get vaccinated is an act of love or not. As much as this may annoy reductionists and lovers of generalizations, every positive moral act must be seen in the concreteness of the existence of each individual person without ever underestimating all the potential aspects involved.

External circumstances and ends include, for example, also religion, to the extent that someone may believe that his faith requires vaccination or treats the vaccine issue with the same epistemological attitude with which a believer treats matters of faith. They include the common good and freedom, insofar as the vaccine issue overlaps or mixes up the individual and the collective good or generates social or justice issues that are greater and/or different from those related to the vaccine itself. I will deal with external circumstances that do not pertain to the order of ends in the fourth conceptual part of this work, which is already complete and available in a volume that enjoys a special scientific and narrative autonomy.[35]

3.3. Internal Institutional and Non-Institutional Circumstances

Among the circumstances internal to the vaccine, we need to distinguish the institutional ones from the non-institutional ones. In fact, anti-Covid vaccines are not a substantial issue that belongs freely, so to speak, to science and civil society. Discussing vaccines is not like talking about the opportunity to choose whether to study medicine or philosophy, or whether it is economically and scientifically convenient to try to develop a new type of electric-powered engine.

Covid vaccines are part of a legalized sector of modern civil society, which means that the discourse on the use of one or more specific vaccines does not start from scratch, from the realm of freedom and human inventiveness, but from rules that regulate the production and testing of new drugs and from prior authorizations for marketing by the political authorities responsible for the examination and approval of these drugs. The discussion starts from the decisions and documents of these authorities, which, evaluating the request of a manufacturer, give vaccines a

35 See F. Di Blasi, *The Death of the Phronimos. Faith and Truth about anti-COVID Vaccines* (Phronesis Editore, Palermo, 2021).

very complex frame of reference, full of conditions and limits of application and use.

Our object of study, therefore, is not simply the anti-Covid vaccine, as an idea for a new entrepreneurial activity or for a new Hollywood movie (or even as a drug in an unregulated, purely imaginary, or primitive, social scientific context). Our object of study is every single Covid vaccine exactly as it has been authorized by the relevant authorities and agencies that have the legal and political power to do so. The study of the vaccine circumstances therefore starts from the reference of the regulatory framework offered by these authorities and agencies. For this institutional regulatory framework, I will refer mainly to the agencies responsible for the United States and Europe: respectively, the U.S. Food & Drug Administration (FDA) and the European Medicines Agency (EMA). Occasionally, I will also refer to other U.S. and European government agencies.

It is essential to understand that the analysis of the circumstances of vaccines through the regulatory framework of the relevant agencies, while focusing on a subject that pertains to drug science, belongs to law and not to science. The processes of government agencies are not the processes of science but of law. Pharmaceutical companies are repositories of drug science, but they produce and test new drugs according to precise rules and regulations and, when they believe they have a product capable of passing the next regulatory filter, they fill out applications for the agencies in charge according to specific legal rules. The decisions of government agencies are therefore based on regulatory criteria and protocols and are not comparable to scientific studies. They are important because they have legal value and not because they make a contribution to science. The arguments used must be transparent and verifiable as in all legal procedures. If agencies make mistakes or do not act according to the rules that govern their processes, they don't have to merely withdraw a flawed scientific essay from a journal (as a scholar would do), but they are also accountable to the political community under the rules that govern their criteria and conduct.

After their conception, which occurs as a result of the embrace between public subsidies and the business potential of pharmaceutical companies, anti-Covid vaccines complete their gestation in a complex legal womb, relating, for example, to safety in production and testing. Their birth certificate into the market is their authorization or approval by the agencies, with all the specific rules and processes that characterize it. This "birth certificate," the genetic context of the vaccine with respect to its public use, is part of our study and generates specific circumstances of the ethical choice. The fact, for example, that a given authorization process has reduced the normal approval and testing times for a drug automatically becomes an important circumstance that the moral agent will have to take into account. The specific assumptions of this procedural exception will become circumstances to be assessed. Likewise, the exact terms of the authorizations with respect to the administration of the vaccine will be circumstances to be considered.

The study of institutional circumstances is a premise, not a conclusion, with respect to overall ethical analysis, which must also consider non-institutional data. Vaccines exist as an option and an ethical issue because they are somehow authorized, but they remain in themselves a substantial question whose study goes beyond the mere genetic data of a legal nature. Where necessary, and to the extent possible and reasonable, I will therefore have to analyze certain circumstances also in the non-institutional context of the broader and international scientific, political, or legal debate. The same circumstances, or similar circumstances, could in fact take on very different connotations inside and outside of the institutional context.

3.4. Internal Structural, Selective, and Evaluative Circumstances

We must then distinguish three types of circumstances which I will call structural, selective, and evaluative. The first category exists only according to the institutional context, but can also concern the debate on non-institutional sources, the other two can be both institutional and non-institutional.

I define structural internal circumstances as those that depend solely on the intrinsic characteristics of the regulatory context of the authorizations of anti-Covid vaccines. I call them structural because they concern the regulatory structure in which the vaccine object comes into the world as a possible object of choice for both politics and individuals. These circumstances concern, as I mentioned earlier, the constitutive conditions of the authorizations and the way in which they become relevant for the agent. For example, knowing that there has been an emergency authorization involving an exception to the normal safety parameters of a drug or vaccine, or the fact that conditions for authorization are the absence of alternatives or the reduction of hospitalizations. These are circumstances that citizens must know before choosing whether to get vaccinated; with respect to these circumstances, research, trials, and therapies outside government agencies and independent of them and of pharmaceutical companies could have a major impact. These structural circumstances, therefore, exist only by virtue of the emergency regulatory context of vaccines, do not concern the specific features of their administration, and can also be assessed according to elements external to those provided by the agencies in charge.

Internal selective and evaluative circumstances, on the other hand, are circumstances that would exist even if there was no starting legal context to deal with. However, they are an integral part of the legal context and must therefore be addressed in detail in that context before addressing them outside of it. Structural circumstances answer the question: "When and under what conditions is it legitimate for a Covid vaccine to be put on the market?" The selective and evaluative ones answer the question: "Given that a vaccine is available on the market, who can use it and when?"

The circumstances that determine the applicability of the vaccine to certain categories of subjects (of a certain age, of a certain sex, with certain pathologies, etc.) are selective. I have called them selective for the simple fact that they initially select the people to whom a certain vaccine can be given. Instead, I have called evaluative those internal circumstances which normally require consideration only when the vaccine is selectively applicable (use of different vaccines, adverse reactions, degree of protection, duration, unknown risks, etc.).

In reality, these two categories of circumstances are very much intertwined and often need to be evaluated together. However, there is a logical sequence in place, such that the selective criterion precedes the evaluative one. If a vaccine, for example, cannot be administered to anyone under the age of 18, then any other vaccine assessment will be useless for those under the age of 18. For those over the age of 18, on the other hand, other arguments related to the circumstances that I have called, in fact, evaluative will be triggered. In my analyses, I will constantly deal with evaluative aspects in the context of selective circumstances because it is impossible to do otherwise and because it is more correct, even epistemologically. However, it is important at least sometimes to address and summarize the evaluative circumstances autonomously and independently of the selective ones.

3.5. Synchronic Aspect and Diachronic Aspect of Circumstances

A very important thing to consider about the circumstances of Covid vaccines is that they can almost never be understood in a static or synchronic sense. The decision to get vaccinated in February 2020 is a different ethical choice than the decision to get vaccinated in September 2021. The decision to authorize the emergency use of an anti-Covid vaccine in December 2019 is a different ethical choice than the decision to allow the emergency use of the same vaccine in December 2021. The circumstances, every circumstance, must be considered in its diachronic value.

This discourse applies above all to circumstances of a legal or institutional nature. If, for example, a prerequisite for the emergency authorization of anti-Covid vaccines is the actual existence of a state of emergency characterized by a fatal disease or the fact that hospitalizations need to be reduced, then if the state of emergency ceases and/or deaths and hospitalizations fall within the norm, the emergency authorization ought to be suspended. Let's imagine that, in a certain state, deaths or hospitalizations from Covid have become equal to or even lower than deaths and hospitalizations due to seasonal flu or other diseases. Why should an emergency authorization be maintained, with the risks it entails, for a disease that is now secondary to others that do not fall within the definition of a state of emergency? Here the diachronic definition and evaluation of the state of emergency becomes fundamental for the ethical and legal decision to keep emergency authorizations in force.

The synchronic analysis, on the other hand, is legally crucial to assess the correctness of the assessments and decisions of the agencies in charge. I do not think anyone has doubts about the state of emergency existing in December 2019, but, for example, there could be doubts about the authorization of the vaccine for some categories of people at a time when absolutely nothing relevant or decisive was known about these categories for the purpose of emergency use of the vaccine. Consider, for example, the extension of some vaccines to the age group from 12 to 15 years. Was there really a pandemic emergency for these people with a significant risk of fatal disease and excess hospitalizations, or was the authorization illegitimately made based on different criteria? Were there sufficient studies to assess the risks and benefits?

Let's move from legal considerations to substantive ones for the individual. Let's think about the assessment of the risks of contagion and serious illness. If the risk statistically increases or decreases, the ethical relevance of that risk will change accordingly, making the choice to get vaccinated respectively easier or more difficult. We can also think that the more time passes, the more the risk of contagion or serious illness decreases for the individual because, at least within certain limits, in a social context characterized by a very contagious viral infection, the fact of staying healthy can serve diachronically as an index showing a robust constitution and a strong immune system, or simply the taking of effective and optimal preventive measures.

Of course, these are only simplified examples of the kind of diachronic reasoning which might affect the assessment of relevant ethical circumstances. In the following, I will try to highlight the importance of the diachronic aspect whenever it will be useful to do so. The basic concept that I want to highlight here is that there is not a single ethical choice relating to the vaccine, neither by the community, through its own legal and political authorities, nor by the individual. The authorities must continuously make new choices, with diachronically updated criteria. And those who have doubts about vaccines will have already made many different ethical choices in this regard and must always reassess their criteria diachronically to understand if the choice they made in the past is still reasonable compared to the new situations and new data available.

3.6. Geographical Aspect of Circumstances

Another aspect that has a huge influence on the assessment of circumstances is geography. Circumstances change in many ways according to location, and this is a fact that should be taken into account more in vaccine studies (or better communicated to the community). Of course, by geographic aspect I do not only mean the one related to different states or regions but also the one related to different environments and to interaction with certain territories.

A person living in the country or in the Midwest does not have the same risk of contagion as a person living in a New York apartment building. Each person, in general, must contextualize the choice to get vaccinated with respect to the territorial or geographical environment in which he or she lives. If it is an environment where social interactions are naturally spaced out and controllable, then the choice to get vaccinated will be more difficult to sustain. Work or social commitments also greatly affect these assessments. Those who live in the countryside may be exposed to greater risks because, for example, they have to travel a lot by plane, or because they work in a hospital in the nearby town. Of course, the risk level of the specific territory must be assessed. If the epidemic is virtually non-existent in a certain city or county or region, the choice of the vaccine becomes very difficult to justify or vice versa.

While writing this book, I have obviously read, studied, and consulted many vaccine-related studies. One thing that struck me about some of them is the unreasonable disproportion between the number of subjects involved and the enormous territorial extension of reference. I am thinking, for example, of a study on about 2,000 children that allowed the extension of the use of the Pfizer vaccine to the 12-15 age group in America and Europe. About 1000 children received the vaccine and 1000 the placebo. I'll go back to this in more detail later. These children were certainly monitored very closely throughout the study, but where did they come from? Where did they live? Did they reasonably represent the entire American and European population? Were those who got infected from high-risk or low-risk areas? Did they go to the disco or the countryside after receiving the vaccine? And, respectively, was it those who received the vaccine or those who received the placebo who went to the disco or to the countryside? Were they a sufficiently diverse group to evaluate the vaccine with respect to a population of about one billion people scattered in such different and distant territories?

3.6.1. Donating Vaccines to African Countries?

I would like to give another example of the importance of the geographical aspect which gives me pause. There is much talk for now (and with good reason) of selfishness and solidarity concerning the enormous availability of vaccines in rich countries compared to poor ones. Some states are actually planning to donate millions of doses to African countries.

Some scandalmongers say these donations are forthcoming because a lot of inventory is about to expire and could not be used in time. Donating them would be a way, for the politicians who purchased them, to transform a failure into a noble gesture. Other scandalmongers say that the urge to donate will slow down or decrease now that it has been discovered that expiration dates can simply be changed by moving them by three months.[36] Then there are the AstraZeneca vaccines, which Europe wants to donate because Europeans—after suspicious deaths and new indications limiting the vaccine to people under 50—no longer want to use them. For us they could be dangerous, and we don't like them anymore, so let's give them to the poor. Of course, these are

36 See "FDA In Brief: FDA Authorizes Longer Time for Refrigerator Storage of Thawed Pfizer-BioNTech COVID-19 Vaccine Prior to Dilution, Making Vaccine More Widely Available," May 19, 2021, URL: https://www.fda.gov/news-events/press-announcements/fda-brief-fda-authorizes-longer-time-refrigerator-storage-thawed-pfizer-biontech-covid-19-vaccine; FDA, "Fact Sheet for Healthcare Providers Administering Vaccine," Last Update September 22, 2021, URL: https://www.fda.gov/media/144413/download: "Cartons and vials of Pfizer-BioNTech COVID-19 Vaccine with an expiry date of May 2021 through February 2022 printed on the label may remain in use for 3 months beyond the printed date as long as approved storage conditions between -90ºC to -60ºC (-130ºF to -76ºF) have been maintained."

just rumors that have no relevance in scientific discourse, but it is also true that politics certainly does not shine these days for its honesty and transparency. Among the thousand reasons behind some noble decisions, some less noble ones are often hidden.

In fact, the very idea of solidarity with poor states arises here from an original sin called "vaccine nationalism": that is, from the phenomenon whereby the richest countries have tried in every way to get favorable contracts with the manufacturers for obtaining reserved or exclusive doses of vaccines to the detriment of other countries. Of course, doing so has also resulted in a rise in the prices of vaccines because the exclusivity costs money.

> "The response to vaccine nationalism has been the creation of the COVAX Facility, an international partnership that aims to financially support leading vaccine candidates and ensure access to vaccines for lower-income countries."[37]

The solidarity of COVAX is a facade solidarity. It is an attempt to patch up the embarrassing nakedness of the rich states. Either way, that's not what I wanted to dwell on. I wanted to focus on the idea itself of donating vaccines to African countries. It sounds like a noble gesture, but does it make sense? The fact is that in Africa, for mysterious reasons that many are wondering about, the epidemic is virtually absent.[38] In many African

---

37 See S. Halabi, A. Heinrich, S. B. Omer, "No-Fault Compensation for Vaccine Injury — The Other Side of Equitable Access to Covid-19 Vaccines," *The New England Journal of Medicine*, December 3, 2020, 383, e125, DOI: 10.1056/NEJMp2030600.

38 See, e.g., M. Senthilingam "Covid-19: Why Africa's Pandemic is Different," *BMJ*, Published October 19, 2021, 375: n2512, doi:10.1136/bmj.n2512; A. Winning, "Puzzled scientists seek reasons behind Africa's low fatality rates from pandemic," Reuters, September 29, 2020, URL: https://www.reuters.com/article/us-health-coronavirus-africa-mortality-i-idUSKBN26K0AI; UN News, "COVID cases surging in Africa at fastest rate this year, but deaths remain low,"

(continued on the next page)

countries, it is impossible to speak of a pandemic state of emergency. If in the United States or in Europe we had had the same number of cases as Africa, there would have been no authorizations for the emergency use of vaccines. So why should we give someone vaccines when their situation would make their use illegal or immoral in our countries? Unless what's behind it is not nobility, but racist utilitarianism. We give them vaccines that we, in their condition, would not take, because in this way they will not infect us if ever a serious epidemic breaks out among them. According to this reasoning, the lives of Africans are less important; they are second-class people, inferior beings. The risk-benefit ratio of vaccines for them should be evaluated, not with respect to their health, but with respect to ours (a bit like one does today with the vaccination of children).

On October 15, 2021, to give a concrete example, President Biden announced the donation of 17 million doses of the Johnson & Johnson vaccine to the African Union during a meeting with the President of Kenya.[39] Of the previous American donation of 50 million doses, Kenya had received about 2.8 million. I don't know how many it has received of this additional donation, but let's focus for a moment on this African state. It has more than 55 million inhabitants, slightly fewer than Italy. As of October 15, 2021, the day of the meeting with Biden, it had had a total of 251,669 cases of Covid and 5,202 deaths since the beginning of the pandemic. The day before, October 14, it had had 186 new cases and 4 deaths. It is also surrounded by states with similar if not lower numbers. Italy, as of October 15, 2021, had had a total of 4,709,753 cases and 131,461 deaths. The day be-

---

December 14, 2021, URL: https://news.un.org/en/story/2021/12/1107882.

39 See, e.g., Z. Kanno-Youngs, "Biden Promotes Vaccine Donation in Meeting With Kenya's President," *The New York Times*, 14/10/2021, URL: https://www.nytimes.com/2021/10/14/us/politics/biden-kenya-kenyatta-ethiopia.html.

fore, October 14, Italy had had 2,666 new cases and 40 deaths. Italy is surrounded by European states with similar or higher numbers.

Now, if we consider that the normal seasonal influenzas in Italy easily reach 4 or 5 million infections and cause between 20 and 50 deaths a day (especially among subjects over 65),[40] it must be deduced that the current situation in Italy has already returned to normality. Kenya's numbers do not even deserve to be included in the statistics of a pandemic. The point is that if we (in Europe or the US) had Kenyan numbers, any emergency vaccine clearance would be illegal. And it would be illegal because it is immoral to take risks on drugs not approved according to the canons of experimental science in the face of a situation that does not in any way fall within the concept of a state of emergency. So why push a state like Kenya to do something that would be illegal and/or immoral for us to do?

To date, many African states have not declared a state of emergency. Among these is Kenya, which has however distinguished itself for very harsh precautionary measures which have included, for example, a curfew and which are similar to the measures adopted in other states that have instead declared a state of emergency or something similar to it, such as the state of calamity or disaster or health emergency or alert. In Kenya, the formal declaration of a state of emergency would require compliance with certain conditions set by the Constitution, "including its duration and its implementation in a manner that respects constitutional rights and freedoms."[41]

40 I will return specifically to these data elsewhere.

41 See E. Gachenga, Deputy Vice Chancellor, Academic and Student Affairs, Strathmore University, "Should the Kenyan Government Declare a State of Emergency?," URL: https://strathmore.edu/news/should-the-kenyan-government-declare-a-state-of-emergency/.

The measures adopted in Kenya and other African states have generated another emergency relating to human rights and there have even been reports of people killed by the police for some time in implementing anti-Covid measures.[42] In some states, such as Malawi, many restrictions have been opposed on the assumption that the reaction to Covid cannot result in people's starvation and malnutrition.[43] Let's leave aside the theoretical assessments on the political reasons that lead many governments to take advantage of the state of emergency (suspending democracy and respect for individual rights) to dramatically increase their power. Here I want to highlight a much more practical problem: namely, that in many states, due to their specific territorial conditions, anti-Covid measures are not justified and risk causing more harm than good. Yet it seems that the only goal of the rich states is to generate the emergency reaction in these states, whatever the consequences, by imposing a blanket vaccination policy at whatever cost.[44]

I will have to return to the utilitarian attitude surrounding various public choices on vaccines at another time. Here it is enough

42 See, e.g., A. Zhu, "Kenya Turns Its Covid-19 Crisis into a Human Rights Emergency," *The New York Review*, July 22, 2020, URL: https://www.nybooks.com/daily/2020/07/22/kenya-turns-its-covid-19-crisis-into-a-human-rights-emergency/; ICNL, "African Government Responses to COVID-19," July 31, 2021, URL: https://www.icnl.org/post/analysis/african-government-response-to-covid-19; PSC Report, "The dangers of states of emergency to combat COVID-19 in Africa," May 26, 2020, URL: https://issafrica.org/pscreport/psc-insights/the-dangers-of-states-of-emergency-to-combat-covid-19-in-africa.

43 See ibid.

44 See, e.g., U.S. Centers for Disease Control and Prevention, "CDC supports Kenya expanding emergency response," Page last reviewed: June 14, 2021, URL: https://www.cdc.gov/globalhealth/stories/2021/cdc-supports-kenya-expanding-emergency-response.html.

for me to point out that the geographical aspect is also crucial for defining the existence or otherwise of the state of crisis and emergency that legally and morally legitimizes the emergency use of vaccines, giving way to more specific assessments concerning them.

3.7. Principles of Analysis

In addition to the typology of the circumstances, I must also clarify in an introductory way what will be the principles and criteria of analysis that I will use for them.

I have already explained the principle to identify the circumstances. I will use both an internal and an external ethical point of view, and I will start with the analysis of the institutional circumstances as they provide the general frame of reference for the whole issue. Now I must focus on the other principles that will be the background to my discourse, from the epistemological method to the use of sources, the legal context, and the analytical and synthetic approach.

3.7.1. Epistemological Method

One of the things that made the ethical evaluation of vaccines more difficult in the current context was the evident discrepancy between the certainties displayed by the political class or mainstream journalism (and seasoned with generic and pseudo-religious references to "science") and the way in which the pandemic has clearly taken the whole world off guard generating, as a potential panacea and in record time, vaccines that seemed to have very few certainties, even for common sense. "Certainty" and "science," abused and mistreated in the political and media forums all over the world, have become the number one enemy of knowledge and moral choice.

Faced with this cultural disaster, the only possible medicine was good epistemology. What truth value do agency sources have? What kind of judgments do they make? What is the value of the reference to science? What disciplines are involved and what in exactly are their experts competent? What can an epidemiologist say scientifically compared to what a physician says? What is the real information about vaccines that we have and what truth value does it have exactly?

In order to return to authentic knowledge and the foundation of a sensible ethical choice, it is necessary to answer these questions. It is necessary to achieve epistemological clarity.

In this context, I will first have to clarify both the scientific status of the disciplines involved and the nature of the judgments of the competent government agencies. The last thing we need is confusion between law and science. A political power that stands as the voice of science or ethics announces disaster. Politics is an animal with hungry instincts for power. Science, culture, and journalism must counterbalance these instincts, not give them assistance towards an enlightened, authoritarian, and absolutist ethical state.

I will then have to analyze—in a meticulous way, when necessary—the truth value, both legal and scientific, of each relevant statement relating to each vaccine contained in the official documents of the agencies endowed with authorization powers. This is a liberating and cathartic activity, necessary even for scientists, to be able to rediscover themselves after so much abuse, even to their detriment, of the "truths" of science. Such a detailed analysis, even if it served no other purpose than this, to recover objectivity and serenity of judgment for the insiders, would still be useful for its redemptive and pedagogical value, and to avoid confusion and similar abuses in the future.

The need to clarify these aspects in an introductory way was not the result of those preparatory and abstract reflections that, like any good scholar, I made on the structure and themes of the book before starting to write it. Rather, it forced itself upon me when addressing the circumstances that I called structural and institutional and, subsequently, when analyzing the specific internal circumstances of specific vaccines. I decided, therefore, to respect its original inspiration and immediacy, and to leave the general analysis of these aspects right there, in the paragraphs of the next two chapters where they were born spontaneously for logical and narrative needs. The alternative was to make it the subject of an introductory chapter on its own, abstracted from the live analysis of vaccines, but it would have been unnecessarily heavy and much less interesting.

I will repeat this one more time in a more direct way. One of the most important methodological principles of this book consists in basing the truth criteria of ethical choice on the recovery of an adequate epistemological sense of the available information concerning vaccines. Epistemology reveals the meaning and scope of technical information on vaccines, making it possible to evaluate them ethically. From this point of view, the method that I will follow in the next chapters will be to summarize, for each relevant circumstance of each vaccine, the technical criteria that the agencies offer us as indications for the choice, and to highlight their epistemological aspects and ethical consequences. I will offer, for each circumstance treated, summary tables: tables on the technical indications of the vaccines and epistemological and ethical tables on those same indications. All these tables, of course, only constitute an aid (never exhaustive) for moral conscience, as they cannot in any way replace the agent's concrete assessments in the here and now of his choice.

A mention of the basic epistemological questions that will accompany us in the next chapters may be useful.

One concerns the scientific and epistemological sense of the evaluation of the risks and benefits of vaccines. Understanding how such an assessment can take place in general is essential for addressing the specific circumstances of vaccines. However, it is only from the analysis of specific circumstances that we seriously realize what it means and implies. Therefore, the introduction to the topic that I will make in the chapters on structural institutional circumstances will show its true face and potential only in the following treatment on selective and evaluative institutional circumstances. The topic of risk assessment also requires some epistemological premises regarding the object and method of medicine and epidemiology. In the immediately following chapters, therefore, I will also have to do this briefly: explain the scientific status of medicine and epidemiology.

Another crucial epistemological question that will be recalled and analyzed in detail in the following chapters and volumes, and which will be the background to the analysis of the individual circumstances, concerns the meaning and the way in which each single anti-Covid vaccine and each single aspect and application of it can be considered experimental or *experimented*, or the sense in which they can be considered the fruit of experimental science as opposed to being in the testing phase. Also in this case, I will first have to provide the general sense of the question and postpone full understanding to the detailed analyses of the individual circumstances.

In Italian, when we say "experimental vaccines" we mean, simply speaking, vaccines that are still in the testing phase, and which cannot therefore be defined as the finished product of a scientific method capable of verifying scientific theories and hypotheses. If a drug is experimental, the patient must use it voluntarily knowing that he is taking part in a clinical trial. In this respect, there has been a heated debate in Italy between the pro-government mainstream narrative that has always tried to argue that anti-Covid vaccines were no longer "experimental" (but already "experimented" or tested) and the alternative narrative that has always maintained that instead they were "experimental" since they were placed on the market before the end of the trials envisaged by the ordinary drug protocols (which generally take five years). Having written this text in two languages, it was easier for me to write according to this Italian semantic convention. Therefore, whenever I refer to "experimental vaccines" or drugs I will always mean this term in the sense of products in the testing phase.

Besides this, other epistemological issues concern the presence and value of studies in conflict of interest or not independent; definitional difficulties that imply uncertainty and imprecision in the studies; contradictory indications between different agencies regarding the same reference studies; references to uncertain or impossible evaluations; contradictions of some indications; use of ambiguous formulas; and the groundlessness of some criteria for authorizations.

3.7.2. Approach to Official Documents and Information

A person might know all that is relevant to know about a certain possibility of action and still decide to do wrong, as does the thief, who knows perfectly well that what he takes is not his and takes it anyway. Knowledge is a necessary premise of the ethical choice, but does not determine its outcome. If knowledge were enough to make one choose well, there would be only ignorant people, not bad people.[45] From a cognitive point of view, however, there is no doubt that the theoretical goodness of the ethical choice is directly proportional to the goodness of the information available. For this reason, it is ethically important to give people all the relevant information so that they can consciously decide how to *regulate* themselves (a splendid term, at least in Italian, which indicates the deepest meaning of moral autonomy, that is, ultimately giving oneself ruling authority over one's actions).

With respect to the need and the ethical duty to provide people with adequate information, I have adopted a specific methodological principle. In my detailed study of specific vaccines, I approached the documents of the competent agencies, the FDA and the EMA, according to subsequent and potential levels of in-depth analysis.

45 Which in itself is one of the most fascinating themes of fundamental ethics ever since it was born with Socrates.

I started with data that are easily available online because those that cannot be found online, or that cannot be found easily, are clearly not among the information that the FDA and EMA consider important to the public. I then divided the information available into three categories

a) Information for end users

   First of all, there are those aimed at end users (the general public), that is, people who can or must receive vaccines. This information can be found in leaflets or factsheets made especially for these people, but also in various pages of FAQs and general presentation of vaccines.

b) Information for operators and professionals

   Then there is the specific information for operators or professionals (a smaller audience) who have to administer the vaccines, contained in other package leaflets.

c) Information for the experts

   Finally, there is information for the knowledgeable public, contained in the technical documents relating to authorizations, changes to authorizations, updates, and product information. These are the documents that are part of the legal administrative procedure of vaccines, those containing their "birth certificate," so to speak, and their bill of good health.

This triple division of relevant information, which in itself seems logically correct to me, is more easily found on the FDA website, which from this point of view appears to be better set up than that of EMA.

Since mine is an ethical analysis that concerns the choices of the end user, it is important for me to follow the opposite path from that which an expert on the subject would follow, who would first of all look at the most fundamental documents regarding the question: from initial authorization up to the last updated product information. In contrast, I am more interested in starting from (simplified) information for the general public, then moving on to (simplified but more detailed) information for the narrower public of healthcare professionals and, finally, when necessary, turning to the complete and technical information of the administrative authorization procedure.

I have to look at things from the point of view of those who try to understand how to regulate themselves and who, by going to the websites of the agencies, try to get adequate information. Naturally, those who do so would first look at the information addressed explicitly to them, then at the information addressed to healthcare professionals and, thirdly, if they still had doubts, they would try to identify and study the more technical documents.

Following this cognitive path of the interested public, or of the ethical subject who acquires information, my analysis will also highlight the clarity and completeness of the information in the first category, but also its consistency with the information in the second and third categories.

My analysis will always start from the FDA documents, also because the EMA decisions on vaccines always follow the FDA decisions. Therefore, I will also highlight the consistency between the decisions and information provided by the FDA and by the EMA regarding the same vaccines and specific aspects of them.

On other methodological criteria relating to sources, I will return specifically, when necessary, in the chapters dedicated to individual circumstances. For example, with respect to the data of seasonal influenzas, I adopted as a methodological criterion that of not using sources after 2018 because I found that, after the start of the controversy over the pandemic, many scholars and agencies began to "interpret" previous data to try to diminish the severity of seasonal influenzas. The reason is that the comparison with seasonal influenzas has led many to question the real state of the coronavirus emergency, at least after the first wave of deaths between 2019 and 2020. Is the current Covid emergency truly greater than the emergency of past seasonal influenzas? Unfortunately, this question is best addressed by looking only at pre-pandemic sources, because subsequent ones are too steeped in what scientific debate calls bias or prejudice.

3.7.3. Legal Approach

I have already highlighted the importance of the legal approach, also concerning the importance of epistemologically distinguishing legal decisions and assessments from purely scientific conclusions.

Here I must clarify that, for me, the legal question also integrates a precise methodological approach to the theme of the book. In fact, I believe both that the ethical importance of the legal aspects surrounding the Covid vaccine issue is greatly underestimated and also that everyone (both the experts and the general public) gets much too confused about what belongs to science and what belongs to the law. This is neither good for science nor for the law. It is no coincidence that the law, with respect to the ethical evaluation of vaccines, is stronger when it is fully aware of itself.

Let me explain. As I will clarify later, one of the key aspects of the law is that you don't mess with it. An expert may be more relaxed about saying what he thinks about a certain matter as long as the law stays in the next room, but when the law walks in and asks him to put his opinions in writing for a court trial or a contract, the expert will think much longer and much better about what he can really say regarding his "science." In this respect, for example, what a pharmaceutical company writes in a contract with the European Union is worth much more than a thousand FAQs and a thousand documents that do not imply direct responsibility. If the contract is secret, there is serious cause for concern. When the European Union's weak and short-sighted politicians decided to agree to conceal the contracts they had signed with the pharmaceutical companies from the public, they launched the largest and most destructive bomb possible on people's trust in Covid vaccines. When contracts are written and signed, the science of law gives, with full awareness, the best of itself, and people know it.

Let's see, instead, what happens when the law is unaware. The pandemic has powerfully confronted us with realities that we could have almost ignored before, such as government drug approval agencies. These agencies are like small parliaments which, in certain areas, decide what will be done in the political community. Their procedures are juridical, their choices political, but they are often seen and presented as if they were entities of a mere scientific nature.

And it's not just a decision problem. As we shall see, some evaluations of opportunities, risks, or advantages also have a legal or political nature. Now, if an evaluation of a political nature is approached or presented as if it were of a scientific nature, it is normal that in a context in which everyone observes what is happening, it ends up generating distrust and doubts in the population. When no one cares about what the FDA and EMA do, these things are not noticed and do not cause worry, but when everyone is anxiously observing the reactions of the authorities in an emergency situation, any dysfunction, in one way or another, emerges. The choice, conscious or unconscious, to create or promote an image of the agencies in question as a mere expression of science was another wrong move compared to the distrust that has been generated in many towards anti Covid vaccines.

If the law were fully aware of itself, at the level of the FDA and EMA, it would first eliminate any semblance of conflict of interest with pharmaceutical companies; it would then formally include some legal experts and some politicians both in the decision-making bodies and in the advisory committees of the agencies; finally, it would always clarify, with respect to public health decisions (especially those made in a state of emergency), what are the contributions of the experts and what legal and political profiles have led to the decisions reached, in a similar way to how a Parliament and a Court use the technical appraisals underlying their laws and verdicts. Citizens have more confidence and are more prone to take risks if the authorities speak to them clearly even about unknowns and hopes. But presenting political choices as if they were mere expressions of science is a deception that in one way or another, and to some extent, can only generate mistrust and confusion.

The juridical aspects have a great importance for the moral conscience and, in what follows, I will try to highlight them as well as possible whenever it is appropriate or necessary.

3.7.4. Analytical and Synthetic Approach

The methodological study of the human act based on the object, the circumstances, and the end implies that a good ethical decision cannot be basically made before having specifically evaluated the individual elements, including all relevant circumstances and possible ends. On the negative side, as we already know, there could be exclusionary circumstances or bad ends. In these cases, moral reasoning could be interrupted, making further analysis and evaluation useless. If a vaccine cannot be taken because you are allergic to it, then it is useless to read all the other warnings. If getting vaccinated just to go to the disco is wrong, then, if that was the only end that inclined me toward that decision, I should stop thinking about it. These, however, are exceptions in my discourse as a whole.

The temptation of those who read an analytical text like this, possibly learning many things they did not know before about anti-Covid vaccines, epistemology, and the moral act, could often be to rush too much towards an ethical conclusion while still at the start of the route or midway. In the 100 or 200-meter dash you can immediately run at maximum speed, but from 800 meters onwards, you need strategy. Those who start too fast do not arrive, or they finish last.

I must therefore warn you, that except in special cases of evident exclusionary circumstances, my analyses of the individual circumstances should not be understood in a synthetic way, as if they already wanted to give conclusive indications on the ethical choice regarding the vaccine, but in an analytical way, as part of a process of study and evaluation that can finally put the ethical subject in the position of making an informed choice. The reader must absolutely avoid the temptation to immediately reach definitive and comprehensive conclusions based on partial elements.

This is a mistake that can be made with both the choice to get vaccinated and not to get vaccinated, of course, but which today is more common in the first case due to misinformation (or news manipulation) intended to convince everyone that getting vaccinated is always a good thing. I have no intention of promoting unfounded and reckless prejudices or judgments. My synthetic judgments on the issue of Covid vaccines are few and uncertain, and I will make extremely parsimonious use of them. In some cases, the choice to get vaccinated seems more obvious to me; in other cases, it is the other way around. However, I am not writing this book to convince someone either in one sense or the other. I am writing it to help everyone's conscience to approach the question more correctly and in a well-informed manner, managing to face the doubts and risks of the truth rather than the easy certainties provided by the media or politicians.

I say this and I will repeat it often throughout the book: my work will be above all analytical, to create distinctions, and my satisfaction will consist above all in bringing people and experts back to honesty and to the complexity of the issues. With exceptions, I do not mean, in the abstract, any of the analyses that I will propose of the individual circumstances as decisive with respect to the ethical choice of anyone—in his existential here and now—to get vaccinated or not. The opposite would be for me a very serious logical, epistemological, and ethical error.

Part II

Internal Structural Institutional Circumstances

As anticipated, in this part of the book we must address the specific treatment of the internal circumstances that I have called institutional: that is, of those circumstances that pertain, on the one hand, to the relationship between anti-Covid vaccines and the sole good of health (and which are therefore *internal* with respect to the vaccine object), and, on the other hand, to the regulatory framework that surrounds the authorizations or approvals of such vaccines (which makes them *institutional*).

We will not, however, speak here of all the internal institutional circumstances, but only of those that I have called structural: that is, those that characterize the regulatory framework that allows the vaccine to be placed on the market but which, in themselves, disregard the specific aspects or methods of use of the individual vaccines. These circumstances have a preliminary value with respect to the whole issue and its ethical relevance. Two, in particular, are of architectural importance, so to speak, and will be the subject of specific chapters. I am referring to the uncertainty about the risks or negative effects of anti-Covid vaccines and their emergency or conditional authorizations. With respect to the second, I will also talk about the AstraZeneca case and the (no longer emergency) approval of the Pfizer/Comirnaty vaccine. I will also devote adequate space to the change in the definition of "vaccine" made by the U.S. CDC.

The circumstance of the emergency authorizations has several assumptions that must also be considered as independent circumstances, such as the state of emergency, the lethality of the disease, the efficacy, the risk-benefit ratio, and the absence of alternatives. In this text, I will only be able to briefly mention these elements, which I intend to deal with in more detail in a future volume of the work.

As I said in the previous chapter, the discussion of these circumstances will also be an opportunity for the specific study of some of the methodological, epistemological, and legal principles that I will use in all the volumes of my work for the analysis of all the circumstances of the moral act.

Chapter 4

Uncertainty about the Negative Effects of Vaccines

This chapter initiates the analysis of the specific circumstances of the moral choice relating to vaccines against Covid. More specifically, I will focus on one of the internal circumstances that I have called "structural institutional." This circumstance stems from the fact that the marketing of anti-Covid vaccines has led, due to the urgency of the pandemic, to the alteration of the normal procedure for approving vaccines, generating uncertainty about their risks. The legal specificity of emergency vaccine approvals will be discussed in the next chapter. Here I do not need to address the technical details of such approvals, but only the fact that they involve a considerable reduction in the ordinary time needed for the approval of vaccines.

Before getting to the subject, I must make a brief methodological premise. We already know that talking about the anti-Covid vaccine in general is objectively wrong because there are different vaccines with different characteristics, approvals, actions, risks, and efficacy. This makes the discussion on the circumstances, like that on the object, very ambiguous and imprecise if it is dealt with in generalities. For example, a certain vaccine may be more suitable for some individuals and not others, or it may not be authorized for some individuals for whom another is authorized. We will therefore have to address the discourse about circumstances specifically for each vaccine. However, in this chapter, I will pretend for simplicity that there is only one anti-Covid vaccine. The circumstance that I am about to analyze is in fact sufficiently general to apply to all vaccines, and, as already mentioned, it will also provide an opportunity to introduce some methodological principles that concern the analysis of other circumstances as well.

4.1. Uncertainty Recognized in Contracts

The procedures for the approval of drugs and vaccines are provided for by international protocols and, as we all know by now, require sufficient time to ascertain above all any negative effects that might occur in the short, medium, and long term.

Of course, when we speak of "sufficient time" we must not take this expression in the sense of some sort of exact mathematical science. There is no formula that can determine when “time” is “sufficient” to say that a product is safe. The time required by the international protocols is the result of a prudent assessment of a probabilistic nature and of likelihood based on the experience of other drugs. A certain product, however, could be a whole other story, and the future, in these areas of knowledge, remains basically inscrutable. The times of the protocols are therefore a reasonable compromise between the scientific community and the law, in the sense that if those times are respected, one falls within the parameters of professional diligence and does not incur responsibility (at least, not with respect to the length of the testing times).

In the case of anti-Covid vaccines, the state of emergency has caused the interruption of the ordinary process for the authorization to trade and has therefore brought with it an intrinsic uncertainty about possible negative effects of the products in question and about possible legal liability. This uncertainty has led pharmaceutical manufacturers, where necessary with respect to individual legal systems, to legally protect themselves by declaring, in contracts with states, that they did not know these effects and that they could not be held responsible for them. States consequently accepted responsibility for the unpredictable damage of vaccines in place of pharmaceutical companies. This is an example of this type of contract clause:

> "Purchaser Acknowledgement. Purchaser acknowledges that the Vaccine and materials related to the Vaccine, and their components and constituent materials are being rapidly developed due to the emergency circumstances of the COVID-19 pandemic and will continue to be studied after provision of the Vaccine to Purchaser under this Agreement. Purchaser further acknowledges that the long-term effects and efficacy of the Vaccine are not currently known and that there may be adverse effects of the Vaccine that are not currently known."[46]

This is an objective circumstance on anti-Covid vaccines which implies an unknown about the future, and which is reflected in the rules that surround them, as well as on the legal need to contractually establish the responsibilities of those involved in their use. Subsequently, we will have to see in detail, both in general and with respect to individual selective and evaluative circumstances, how this aspect of uncertainty emerges from the authorization documents and information provided by the competent agencies. This type of circumstance intrinsically requires a risk-benefit assessment which, being based on a bet on the future, cannot by its very nature generate strong epistemological or moral certainties. From the point of view of this circumstance, this ethical choice will always be characterized by a not indifferent intrinsic doubt.

46 Pfizer supply agreement in Europe. The emphasis is mine.

4.2. Logic, Bets, and the Impossible Evaluation of Risks and Benefits

The last aspect I referred to deserves clarification. When I speak of "bets" I do it in a purely logical sense. In the case of drugs or vaccines that have followed the ordinary international protocols, the leaflets (albeit within the generic limits of human science and, therefore, of the research carried out and the protocols in use at a given historical moment) tell us what we risk. Consequently, in taking those drugs or vaccines, we can assess the risks and benefits based on the information contained in the leaflets.

In the case of Covid vaccines, however, the medium and long-term effects (and sometimes even the short-term effects) are not known because the medium and long-term still exist only in the future (and the short-term effects have sometimes not been studied, or not studied enough). Maybe we are very certain of some short-term effects because vaccines have been administered to billions of people and there have been several studies, but with respect to the medium and long-term effects, or to cases not yet studied, we cannot even make objective hypotheses because we do not have data yet; we have no cases; we have no symptoms or correlations' analyses.

As far as we know now, anything and everything could happen with respect to any consequence: tumors, warts, infertility, pointy ears, hooked noses, baldness, or heart attacks. Seriously, it might be that vaccines will not cause any short, medium, or long-term problems (and we all hope so, given the staggering number of people who have already received the vaccines). However, it could also be the case that the most disparate negative effects will occur that no one is even considering now, and that perhaps are not being detected due to the way in which the reporting and/or passive pharmacovigilance system is structured (or being discouraged).

When we approach these vaccines, the doctor will not be able to tell us that there is a certain percentage of probability that, in the medium and long term, we will have a tumor, experience an early heart attack, or become sterile. He will not be able to tell us this for the simple fact that no epidemiological survey can be transmitted to us from the future with a time machine. An assessment of medium and long-term risks is therefore a gamble of which people should be aware. And there is no science that can make this assessment, precisely because there is no science without the object of study, which exists only in the future. I will return shortly in this regard, and in more detail, to the way in which relevant studies of an epidemiological nature take place.

4.3. The Leaflet Objection

All those objections that circulate on TV and in the mass media regarding the fact that other drugs also have contraindications and that we generally do not read their leaflets are illogical and superficial because, in the case of normal drugs, we can trust the ordinary approval processes and advice from doctors (that have read the leaflets). Regular drugs are also tested over the medium and long-term because they are approved after all tests have been completed (which generally takes several years). In this case, however, no one, not even doctors, can make any assessment because the data simply do not yet exist.

Everyone, including physicians, must therefore make a bet on leaflets that have never been written and that no one can know. The question is not why some people are interested in leaflets in this specific case. The question is how even physicians can make a risk assessment in the case of a drug or vaccine that does not have medical information leaflets, or, better, whose leaflets vary from week to week and will be reasonably complete and fully reliable (even with respect to identifying any long-term risks) only in several years, at best.

4.4. The Epistemology of Risk Assessments

As we shall see later, an extremely uncertain panorama emerges from the detailed analysis of the official documents on anti-Covid vaccines. The basic truth is that the data held by the competent authorities (or at least the data that the competent authorities are willing to share with the public) are, in general, not sufficient for reliable assessments.

To me, personally, one of the things that is most stupefying is precisely the claim, which I have just mentioned, of having assessed the unknown or potential risks of anti-Covid vaccines in the face of an evident and total lack of data processing in this regard. In other words, the relevant government agencies promptly state that they have authorized the vaccines based on a benefit-risk assessment that also includes unknown or potential risks. This type of evaluation is in some way a necessary act (psychologically) because, remember, the vaccines in question have been approved by shortening the medium and long-term testing times. Something must also be said about what to expect in the future (so, at least, they seem to think in the agencies).

This, as I have already said, is an aspect that I will analyze in detail later for each vaccine and for each relevant aspect of that vaccine. Let's look at it now, however, in general, from the perspective of the agencies that have to provide answers to the public. Again, it is obvious that these agencies feel like they should also give this type of response. They must tell us whether these hypothetical, possible, or potential risks have been considered and how. They always tell us clearly that these risks have been considered, but what about the how?

Faced with the claim that the unknown risks have been considered, I, who have an epistemological doubt about how they could have done so (given that these risks belong to the future and concern an unprecedented type of product), became particularly curious and started looking for clues in the documents concerning each individual vaccine. As I will show in dealing with the individual vaccines, I have found nothing at all. There is no trace of this type of risk, which they tell us (repeatedly and concerning every relevant aspect of every single vaccine) they have considered.

Now, in the professional and scientific world, when there is no trace of a certain issue in the working documents, we all know what this means; it means that the judgment on it is intuitive in nature and, therefore, unscientific. Science, especially experimental science, is a serious matter. Science comes from the Latin *scire*, which means to know. Scientific knowledge is highly qualified knowledge which, due to the way it is obtained, acquires greater certainty and predictive capacity than other forms of knowledge.[47] Scientific knowledge without theories and supporting data does not exist. And in this case, it is just so, and the documents confirm it. If there were supporting data, it would have been explained and developed somewhere. The agencies' assessment of the risks and benefits of anti-Covid vaccines, at least in the part concerning unknown future risks, is intuitive in nature; it is guesswork, speculation, mere conjecture.

4.4.1. Guesswork and Off-Label Use of Drugs

I don't want to give the wrong impression, however. Guesswork is not erroneous in itself. Sometimes, in life, it is the only thing that can be done. Also, guesswork is not the same for everyone. There is a qualified kind of guesswork, done by people specializing in a certain subject or discipline, and there is the common man's guesswork, in subjects about which we all have similar experience. Every professional uses a bit of guesswork in

---

47 On the meaning of scientific knowledge compared to other forms of knowledge I dwell more particularly in the book *The death of the Phronimos: Faith and Truth about anti-COVID Vaccines* (Phronesis Editore: Palermo, 2021) which, as I said in the introduction, is subsequent to this volume but was published first for reasons of editorial choice, proofreading, and revision.

his work because there are not already elaborated and developed scientific answers for everything. Even guesswork, however, can and must be argued, and anyone who has participated in business meetings with colleagues knows this well. The guesswork needs to be argued even more in the case of shared decisions, precisely because it is not based on reliable scientific data available and must allow for agreement among the professionals involved.

An example of qualified medical guesswork is the off-label use of a drug: that is, the therapeutic use of a drug for situations other than those for which the drug was approved. This is something absolutely normal and accepted in medicine because the professional experience of a doctor—which also includes the knowledge of the chemical and scientific principles of drugs—can assess that a certain drug is what a patient needs, even if this does not fall within the *scientific* indications of the leaflet.

> "Off-label prescribing is when a physician gives you a drug that the U.S. Food and Drug Administration (FDA) has approved to treat a condition different than your condition. This practice is legal and common. In fact, one in five prescriptions written today are for off-label use."[48]

Off-label use also, by definition, includes the experimentation phase of a new drug because this takes place without or beyond its authorization for use. Studies on booster doses of vaccines, for example, have sometimes required authorizations for off-label use of the vaccines (which had not been authorized for this type of doses).[49] Epistemologically, any pharmacological experimenta-

---

48 See AHRQ - Agency for Healthcare Research and Quality, "Off-Label Drugs: What You Need to Know," URL: https://www.ahrq.gov/patients-consumers/patient-involvement/off-label-drug-usage.html.

49 See, e. g., V.G. Hall, V.H. Ferreira, T. Ku, M. Ierullo, B. Majchrzak-Kita, C. Chaparro, N. Selzner, J. Schiff, M. McDonald, G. Tomlinson, V. Kulasingam, D. Kumar, A. Humar, "Randomized trial of a third

(continued on the next page)

tion is based, not on experimental science, which can be developed only after the experimentation has taken place, but on theoretical hypotheses and on qualified guesswork that, with the consent of the patient and sometimes with the authorization of the competent authorities, accepts the risk of the unknowns of the case.

To facilitate the discussion, let's refer to a TV series with which doctors have a love-hate relationship, House. Let's have some fun with this TV show, then, by recalling an episode in which House must answer for his cases to a medical examiner:

> "Examiner: Patient, 62 years old. You prescribed Viagra. I look in vain for the words erectile dysfunction in the notes for Dolores Smith.
>
> House: She had a heart condition.
>
> Examiner: And you ran out of nitroglycerine?
>
> House: She also had low blood pressure. So, nitro would be dangerous. Little blue pills improve blood flow. They're vasodilators. It's why you sometimes get the headaches."[50]

Of course, I don't care about the technical merits of House's answer. It could also be a medical mistake made by the writers. All I care about is the fact that House defended his choice to use a drug outside the parameters of "mainstream science" in its regard. On this, that is, on the epistemological aspects of professional guesswork, the screenwriters were not wrong. Indeed, as

---

dose of mRNA-1273 vaccine in transplant recipients - Letter to the Editor," "Supplementary Appendix," *The New England Journal of Medicine*, vol 385, n. 13, 2021, pp. 1244-1246, published online on August 11, 2021, URL: https://www.nejm.org/doi/full/10.1056/NEJMc2111462: "A notice of approval to conduct the study was also obtained from Health Canada due to off-label use of a third dose of mRNA-1273 vaccine."

50 See House, Season 2, episode 10.

we will see later, they have done better than the FDA and EMA did when it comes to assessing the unknown risks of vaccines.

Let's think more about the epistemology of House's response. He relies on the scientific knowledge of the active ingredients of the two drugs mentioned and of their negative side effects. Nitroglycerin, hypothetically, helps the heart, but damages blood pressure. Viagra is a vasodilator; it helps the heart, but can cause some headaches. A headache for that patient is an acceptable risk; the effect of nitroglycerin on blood pressure is not. Is that true? Were the writers of House right? I repeat, I don't know, and I don't care. I'm interested in the epistemology of this risk-benefit assessment, an assessment which, while implying a guesswork in the off-label use of a drug, is specifically argued.

From an epistemological point of view, the important thing that needs to be understood about this guesswork is that it is based, on the one hand, on the experience of the doctor and his relationship with the patient and, on the other hand, on the scientific knowledge that the doctor has, not of the leaflet, but of the active principles of drugs of which every aspect has been tested and the effects are known. In the case of vaccines against Covid, however, there is a fundamental difference: they are based on a principle or technique never used before and with respect to which, precisely because there is no long-term experience, the whole world questions itself with concern.

This concern is not induced by some category of unbalanced subjects that the fanatical press likes to, disparagingly, call "anti-vaxxers." It arises from the basic operations of human intelligence with respect to the genesis of the current vaccines against Covid-19. In fact, the first institutional trace of this concern is found in the meeting of the Advisory Committee of independent FDA experts that preceded the first emergency authorization in the world, that of the Pfizer/Comirnaty vaccine.

> "The committee discussed potential implications of loss of blinded, placebo-controlled follow-up in ongoing trials including how this may impact availability of safety data to

> support a biologics license application. Some pointed out the importance of long-term safety data for the PfizerBioNTech COVID-19 Vaccine as it is made using a technology not used in previously licensed vaccines."[51]

It is precisely this epistemological technical aspect that perplexes me; and I have searched in vain for plausible arguments about it. How do you argue about still unknown risks of something never experienced before? I don't think it can be done, but I was ready to be proven wrong based on the official documents supporting the vaccines. As I will show in the analysis of specific cases and circumstance, I have not been proven wrong. The FDA and EMA do not provide any plausible arguments in this regard. Their guesswork is therefore unfounded and deceptive. Certainly, it is not the outcome of any science related to medicine.

The only reference to the evaluation of future effects that I found, in the memorandum on the first vaccine approval to which I have just referred, is the following:

> "Potential risks that should be further evaluated include uncommon to rare clinically significant adverse reactions that may become apparent with more widespread use of the vaccine and with longer duration of follow-up (including further evaluation of risk of Bell's palsy and allergic reactions following vaccination), risks associated with vaccination of specific populations such as children younger than 16 years of age and pregnant and breastfeeding women, and whether vaccine-enhanced disease could occur with waning of immunity."[52]

---

51 See FDA, "Comirnaty and Pfizer-BioNTech COVID-19 Vaccine - Emergency Use Authorization (EUA) for an Unapproved Product Review Memorandum," December 11, 2020, URL: https://www.fda.gov/media/144416/download.
52 Ibid.

Scientifically speaking, this mention of potential adverse effects to study and evaluate means very little and is by no means exhaustive. How could it be? We can only deduce, on the one hand, that there were already specific concerns for categories of subjects that, as we shall see, had been excluded from the initial studies, and, on the other hand, that it is known that adverse effects could occur precisely in the long run with the widespread use of the vaccine. If anything, it is worth noting the mention of the possibility that it is the vaccine, in the future, that will somehow potentiate the disease.[53] Here the difference between the discussion among experts, on the one hand, and the propaganda of many politicians and journalists, on the other, is apparent.

From a logical point of view, assessing the future risks of new drugs is only a gamble. Let me add now that I do not think it is a comparable bet to that of playing dice. It is still a type of guesswork based on generally similar experiences by the experts involved. However, it is a kind of guesswork about which it must be clarified, from an epistemological point of view, that it implies a leap in the dark of uncertain and unpredictable dimensions. In fact, it is not based in any way on concrete and specific experiences already made or on drugs whose long-term effects are already known.

This aspect must be specifically emphasized; otherwise we end up, even if sometimes in good faith, deceiving or misleading ourselves and other people. Everyone in life has to take risks at times, and I do not condemn politicians or government agency experts

53 "Vaccine-associated enhanced disease (VAED) occurs when an individual who has received a vaccine, develops a more severe presentation of that disease when subsequently exposed to that virus, compared with when infection occurs without prior vaccination" (N. Crawford, A. Harris, G. Lewis, "Vaccine-Associated enhanced disease (VAED)," *Melbourne Vaccine Education Center*, January 2021, URL: https://mvec.mcri.edu.au/references/vaccine-associated-enhanced-disease-vaed/).

for this. However, people must be treated with maturity and honesty, which includes exposing one's doubts in the face of risky choices. Once upon a time, politicians prayed, even publicly, to make the right choice. Today they try to convince everyone that "science" supports and guarantees their decisions 100%. This is wrong. Epistemologically, in these cases, the prayer is correct; the reference to science is wrong. I must also say that I wouldn't be so firm on this point if it weren't for how the mainstream media, agencies, and political establishment dealt with off-label uses of other drugs by physicians genuinely committed to treating their patients during the pandemic. But I'll have to come back to that at another time.

4.5. Main Epistemological Issues Concerning Vaccines

In general, the epistemological aspects of anti-Covid vaccines concern the value of the data that are the basis of the authorizations and specific indications concerning vaccines. On the one hand, it is a question of assessing whether the data are sufficient or reliable and, on the other, whether they are used correctly. Some data, for example, may have been collected in conflict of interest situations and, in these cases, it is necessary either to question the general reliability of those who propose the data or to request other independent data. Some data may be too small or limited and not reflect sufficient consensus from the scientific community. Some data could be misused.

It is an epistemological problem, for example, to understand on the basis of which data a certain vaccine is recommended (and how) to people of a certain age group or to a certain category of people such as immunocompromised or pregnant women. It is an epistemological problem to understand on the basis of which data a vaccine can be considered experimental, effective, or safe. In these cases, it is not a question of judging the validity or reliability of the data as such, but of evaluating whether the connection between the data used in the premise of line of reasoning and the conclusion of that reasoning is logically correct.

There are some epistemological questions regarding anti-Covid vaccines that have important repercussions on ethical choice, and which I will therefore have to ask myself about specifically for each individual anti-Covid vaccine and for each use of it with respect to individual pathologies or categories of subjects. For example:

1) Concistency of experimental science

Evaluation of the available or presumed knowledge on vaccines (short, medium, or long term) with respect to the parameters of experimental science. When can a theoretical or hypothetical truth be attested in terms of experimental science? Experimental science adds something to purely theoretical science, but this something must be, by the very nature of experimental science, the result of adequate experiments and—within reasonable and epistemologically shareable parameters—conclusive.

2) Degree of scientific certainty

Assessment of the degree of scientific certainty of available or presumed knowledge on these vaccines. Not all information and claims circulating on anti-Covid vaccines have the same degree of scientific certainty. When and to what extent can they be relied upon?

3) Concistency between truth and decisions

Evaluation of the scientific consistency between the truth value of the studies based on the authorizations and recommendations, on the one hand, and the truth content of the authorizations and recommendations, on the other. Scientific studies often precede political and institutional decisions on vaccines by governments and drug agencies. There is no guarantee, however, that the premises are adequate or sufficient for the conclusions.

4) Truth concistency of the assessments set out in the premises

Scientific and truth value of the assessments based on the authorizations and recommendations on anti-Covid vaccines. Any decision on these vaccines presupposes assessments of the available data and of the issues that are a matter of concern. The scientific and truth value of these assessments depend on their consistency with the data and issues, and on the way in which they are argued.

5) Conflicts of interest

Presence and importance of conflicts of interest. Conflicts of interest naturally affect the reliability and, therefore, the truth value of studies, evaluations, and decisions. This is why legal systems have specific rules in this regard. Conflicts of interest must always be identified, and their relevance must be assessed with respect to the contexts and situations they affect.

6) Judgments on efficacy

Scientific and truth value of judgments on efficacy. The efficacy of anti-Covid vaccines is a premise of their own emergency authorization, as well as of the technical and ethical judgments on them. Efficacy is one of the aspects that has most characterized the public debate on these vaccines, but it is also one of the aspects of them that seemed more uncertain and fluid. It is important to question the scientific and truth-bearing basis of both the initial synchronic judgment on the efficacy of vaccines and the constantly changing opinions on their efficacy in a diachronic sense.

7) Judgments on safety

Scientific and truth value of safety judgments. What has been said about efficacy also applies to the safety of anti-Covid vaccines, which has been characterized by constant updating of contraindications and legal provisions (both restrictive and extensive) on their use.

8) Risk benefit assessments

Scientific and truth value of risk-benefit assessments. These assessments are perhaps the most important with respect to both the emergency authorizations of anti-Covid vaccines and the continued use of them. The structure of epistemological reliability in both a synchronic and diachronic sense must be carefully evaluated.

9) Consultation with the doctor

Gnoseological assumptions of a consultation with a physician. Consultation with a doctor depends on the available knowledge about anti-Covid vaccines. It is scientifically unfounded to postpone the decision to administer these vaccines to a doctor's consultation when there is nothing scientific that the doctor can say or evaluate with respect to them. It is important to check whether the competent authorities refer to a consultation with a doctor in a scientifically acceptable way with respect to the specific aspects of the vaccines.

10) Indications on drugs

Coherence, consistency, or contradiction of the indications. The indications on anti-Covid vaccines must be the conclusion of correct and verifiable premises. The degree of certainty and reliability of the indications themselves in terms of conclusions depends on the relevant premises. As regards the indications, therefore, if we want to be able to evaluate their degree of reliability, we must ask ourselves about the premises and the reasoning that justify them.

11) Contraindications and adverse effects

Coherence, consistency, or contradiction of contraindications. What has been said about the indications applies, of course, also to the contraindications.

12) Presuppoitions of booster or additional doses

Scientific and truth value of the assessments and assumptions of booster or extra doses. The intense debate on extra or booster doses is particularly interesting, from an epistemological point of view, both with respect to these doses themselves, and because it is recent and revitalizes the fundamental issues regarding anti-Covid vaccine decisions in general.

All these epistemological questions, and others connected, require a specific treatment in relation to each vaccine and to each relevant circumstance of it, also highlighting the consequences on the moral choice. I will focus particularly on the issue of vaccine testing after carefully addressing the epistemological status of medicine and epidemiology.

4.6. Medicine, Epidemiology, and Knowledge of Adverse Effects

It is also important to understand how the adverse or negative effects of a drug are studied or discovered. This is done through epidemiological studies. But how do these studies work? The frequent references to "science" during this period are in and of themselves deceptive and lead people to think that the adverse effects of a drug can be deduced with certainty from some kind of equation, or some known scientific truth. It suggests that "scientists" may know or predict the adverse effects of a vaccine based on their alleged abstract scientific knowledge of reality, or that television virologists (this new category of showbiz characters) actually have anything relevant to say. Nothing could be further from the truth.

First of all, it must be understood that epidemiology is not medicine. As I will never tire of repeating, medicine is not science (or knowledge) of the universal, but of the particular. It is the science that has as its object the patient, every single patient. The closer medicine gets to its proper object, the less it allows for abstraction and generalization. This is the crucial epistemological aspect of medicine, which is why physicians often express their anger toward other scholars by saying "they don't have their scrubs on." What they mean is that other kinds of scholars don't know what it means to actually treat a patient or to help him heal because, unlike physicians, they work on abstractly isolated aspects of reality. Particular reality is not reducible to universal formulas and always presents a richness and unpredictability that catches any abstract knowledge off guard. One can be abstractly sure that a certain drug is effective against a certain virus or bacterium or that it cures a certain pathology, but one can never be abstractly sure that this is the drug that a certain patient needs at that precise moment in which his or her doctor must make a decision.

It is also necessary to consider the complexity of reality. For a certain patient, a drug can become a poison and a poison can become a drug. Even smoking might be good for some patients.[54] Sometimes a drug may not be indicated per se for a certain pathology, but if combined with another drug and used as part of a particular therapy, it could have positive effects. These are things

54 There are cases, it seems, in which certain psychological benefits of smoking can outweigh, for some patients, the physical harm that could derive from it.

that the physician notices before the scientist does, because they arise from the relationship with reality rather than from the process that abstracts from it. I will return to these epistemological aspects of medicine at another moment. Now I must instead turn specifically to epidemiology.

Epidemiology is fundamentally statistical. It is a discipline dominated by mathematical models. This is an obvious epistemological fact for a philosopher, and it is the reason why there cannot be an epidemiological study of future events. Statistics are based only on what has already happened. Many have probably never wondered, for example, what the basic scientific foundations of the lists of carcinogenic foods are. Simple, they are statistical observations, over the years and on as many people as possible, of the carcinogenic effects of a certain food (hoping, of course, to be able to sufficiently isolate the effects from those of other foods and/or of other relevant circumstances, which is really not easy to do).

There is basically no abstract scientific formula that allows us to conclude with certainty that a food is carcinogenic, just as there is no abstract formula that allows us to predict all the possible negative effects of a new drug before somehow monitoring its effects. The human being is so complex and unpredictable that any hypothesis, however well based on previous experiences or theories, must finally deal with the statistics of what happens when eating a certain food or taking a certain drug. When a drug is authorized in an emergency, skipping the short, medium, or long-term trials, epidemiology has absolutely nothing scientific to tell us about its potential future adverse effects. For philosophers who have some basic notion of gnoseology (and of the branch of gnoseology applied to science which is called epistemology), this is a truism.

Still, since in this book I am not addressing primarily my fellow philosophers but people who have doubts about vaccines, I will explain this fundamental trait of epidemiology by referring to one of the main agencies involved in the current debate and in choices on vaccines, the U.S. Centers for Disease Control and Prevention (CDC). Over the years, this agency has developed its own epidemiology manual which is also offered as an online self-study course option for anyone wishing to acquire the basics of this discipline. Let's see, then, if the statistical nature of epidemiology emerges clearly from the CDC manual.

> "What is Epidemiology?
>
> Epidemiology is the method used to find the causes of health outcomes and diseases in populations. In epidemiology, the patient is the community and individuals are viewed collectively. By definition, epidemiology is the study (scientific, systematic, and data-driven) of the distribution (frequency, pattern) and determinants (causes, risk factors) of health-related states and events (not just diseases) in specified populations (neighborhood, school, city, state, country, global). It is also the application of this study to the control of health problems."[55]
>
> "The Epidemiologic Approach:
>
> As with all scientific endeavors, the practice of epidemiology relies on a systematic approach. In very simple terms, the epidemiologist:
>
> - **Counts** cases or health events, and describes them in terms of time, place, and person;
> - **Divides** the number of cases by an appropriate denominator to calculate rates; and

55 See CDC, "Epidemiology - What is Epidemiology?," URL: https://www.cdc.gov/careerpaths/k12teacherroadmap/epidemiology.html.

- **Compares** these rates over time or for different groups of people."[56]

For an analytical mind like mine, the first line of the proposed definition is perhaps the most significant because it reveals how an epidemiologist sees himself today. The introduction by the CDC does not claim the scientific autonomy of a discipline, but of a method. Epidemiology is basically a method of calculation: counting, dividing, and comparing.

The second revealing note is the departure from medicine. The patient is the community. One does not look at the individual, but at the community. This is obvious for the statistical calculation, and also in line with the etymology, which comes from the Greek words *epi* (on), *demos* (people) and *logos* (rational discussion). From a logical point of view, this approach conceptually disconnects epidemiology from medicine. If it is a population-related calculation method, then it can be used for anything that is relative to the population as a whole, including terrorist phenomena, domestic violence, or statistical numbers of murders and natural disasters. If the CDC specializes in a calculation method related to population, it is obvious that the Government may ask it to calculate any phenomenon of interest that affects the population, even if in itself unrelated to medicine. Some will think that I am being ironic and that it is not serious to make fun of a science as important to medicine as epidemiology by reducing it to a mere method of calculating any phenomenon relating to the population. I would never have allowed myself to be ironic in such matter. I mean, I knew and always thought that epidemiology was basically statistics, but I would never have allowed myself to say it so bluntly and with these kinds of examples if the

56 See CDC, "Lesson 1: Introduction to Epidemiology. Section 5: The Epidemiologic Approach," URL: https://www.cdc.gov/csels/dsepd/ss1978/lesson1/section5.html.

CDC hadn't done so before I did. All the examples I have just given, from 9/11 terrorism to domestic violence, I have taken from the introductory page on epidemiology from which I have just cited the definitional notion offered to us by the CDC.

Statistics is an important thing, but knowledge based on statistics has a weaker truth value than real science. Real science tells me that if I build a car or a cell phone a certain way, it will work and have a certain kind of performance. It tells me that under certain conditions of pressure a human being dies. If a statistician tells me that in my factory, for every 100 machines I build, on average, 70 work, I know that I must hire better engineers or stop production. If a statistician tells me that 40% of all divers who dive over 20 meters die, it does not give me any real scientific information on the nature of the effect that diving over 20 meters has on human life.

I do not want to denigrate epidemiology now, which I deeply respect as I do all sectors of human knowledge. I just want to emphasize that the medical knowledge we have of the adverse effects of drugs is weak because it is based, for the most part, on the statistical observation of what happens to those who take them. The leaflets are not written when we understand everything about the adverse effects (when we know their *science*), but when it is reasonably certain (epidemiologically, or, that is, statistically) that those effects occur with a given frequency. The correlation itself between the drug and the adverse effect is not supposed to be ascertained in the sense that its "why" is understood, but in way similar to the procedure in a criminal trial when the event "accident" is materially linked to the event "car" without necessarily knowing yet whether the relevant damage was caused by the driver. Many adverse events of the drugs included in the leaflets are unexplained, or have not yet been explained by science, but are ascertained by a statistical calculation considered to be reliable.

Furthermore, precisely because statistics are not based on understanding why, but rather on "count, divide and compare," it is possible that statistics reaches the wrong conclusions only because it underestimates the relevant data or badly isolates them or underestimates their correlation with other data or events. Imagine, for example, that an epidemiological study shows that a drug hurts, but without having considered its timing of administration with respect to the relevant pathology or the interaction with other drugs in the context of a complex therapy. The study could conclude that the drug hurts when the drug would be great if given at the right time and as part of a broader therapy.[57] The point of observation, selection of data, and isolation of the data from other relevant factors can sometimes cause studies of the same data to go in diametrically opposite directions. Imagine that a certain drug advertised to improve sports or outdoor performance has a proven negative effect on blood pressure but that, overall, it is epidemiologically known that the people who take it are better off. But are they better off because of the chemical effect of that drug or because when they take it, they tend psycho-

57 I am thinking, for example, with respect to Covid-19, of the case of hyperimmune plasma, which is very effective if administered early, when the patient's problem is still the fight against the virus and not the inflammation caused by it. In Italy, for unknown reasons, so-called TV experts, the media, and politics ensured that there was no investment in hyperimmune plasma, discrediting it as a completely useless therapy. The responsibilities of this scientifically unfounded and grossly negligent attitude should be ascertained because, indeed, the early use of this therapy could have saved many lives and facilitated the natural immunity of the population. On this, see the excellent journalistic investigation carried out by the Italian TV broadcast "Le iene," in which they also interviewed Arturo Casadevall, Chair of the Department of Molecular Microbiology and Immunology, Johns Hopkins Bloomberg School of Public Health, and the expert in hyperimmune plasma and Professor of Anesthesiology Michael J. Joyner, of the Mayo Clinic: See *Le iene*, "The news on hyperimmune plasma and monoclonal antibodies," April 27, 2021, URL: https://www.iene.mediaset.it/video/plasma-iperimmune-e-anticorpi-monoclonali_1039930.shtml.

logically to do more sports and outdoor activities? Is it the drug or the outdoor activity that makes them healthier? In the first case, the balancing of risks and benefits would be in favor of the drug; in the second, taking the drug would per se have the only ascertained negative effect on blood pressure.

I now return to my initial doubt by arguing it more precisely. If the effects of a new drug or vaccine are seen through epidemiological studies, the statistics based on these studies can only be calculated *in itinere* (in progress), as the vaccine is tested in the short, medium, and long term. From a scientific point of view, epidemiology cannot tell us absolutely anything about future data on which it has not yet been able to draw up adequate statistics. Furthermore, epidemiology cannot afford any guesswork, because statistics and mathematical models do not allow this type of conjectural judgment, other than "statistical" ones based on past data and experiments. Epidemiology cannot bse itself on guesswork drawn from unprocessed statistics of facts that have never occurred relating to things that have not yet been identified.

On the other hand, epidemiology or not, the weakness of anti-Covid vaccine *science* is clearly seen in its evident and continuous failures in predicting the duration of vaccine efficacy, herd immunity, or the end of the pandemic. True science is always predictive. When science can't predict or fails in its predictions, it's never true science, even though some alleged scientists may scream a lot on television. Alas, the intensity of the televised screams is not an adequate criterion for scientific experimentation nor, fortunately, is it recognized by the scientific community. Scientific models could perhaps be devised to predict (based on vanity and other typical motivations) how much and why certain people will scream when they are on television. But this is indifferent to the scientific approach to anti-Covid vaccines and goes beyond the limits and interests of this book. Let's face it, statistically the best scholars don't appear on television these days, or they don't appear very frequently or very willingly

4.7. Experimental or Non-Experimental Vaccines?

Let us now return to the epistemological question of experimentation. Here, with reference to the circumstance of the medium and long-term (but also, in some cases, short-term) unknowns, a huge mass disinformation campaign was carried out by playing on the idea that anti-Covid vaccines were not experimental. This campaign was certainly conducted in bad faith by many experts, by many individuals with institutional duties and by many journalists. Others have carried it out simply out of intellectual mediocrity or some kind of fanaticism. Evidently, it was thought that the (alleged) anti-vaxxers were effectively using the argument that the vaccines were experimental. The team order was therefore to try to make them ridiculous by explaining that these vaccines, in reality, are not experimental at all.

Generally, it is we philosophers who risk dwelling so much on certain concepts that we lose contact with reality or fall into useless nominalistic disputes. In this case, on the other hand, due to the fanaticism with which people approach the topic of anti-Covid vaccines, the nominalistic and useless disputes were carried out by many unsuspected people who have nothing (or shouldn't have anything) to do with philosophy.

If we want to be serious people and avoid nominalistic games, the first thing we must ask ourselves about this dispute is what is the relevant information to give to the public. The answer is that the substance of this information is precisely the circumstance that, in the case of these so-called vaccines, the approval protocols have been cut in order to be able to put them on the market quickly. By doing so, products were immediately made available whose potential negative effects are not known, especially in the medium and long term. And even their effectiveness is not fully known. The effects will be monitored—and therefore detected, analyzed, and evaluated—*in itinere*, in progress. Whatever the name we attribute to this circumstance to inform the public, the important thing is that this name is able to convey the information correctly and unambiguously.

> *Question*: "With respect to what can it be said that these vaccines have been tested?"
>
> *Answer*: "In general, with respect to a certain short-term efficacy limited to certain categories or groups of subjects and with respect to medium-term data that vary from day to day."
>
> *Question*: "Compared to what can we say that these vaccines are still in the experimental phase or, more simply, *experimental*?"
>
> *Answer*: "With respect to their overall efficacy in fighting the epidemic, with respect to the categories of people not included in the initial studies, and with respect to their medium and long-term effects."

Now, since this controversy was born in public opinion and concerns the correct information on anti-Covid vaccines, any semantic value of the terms "experimental" and "tested" must be evaluated above all in relation to their ability to correctly convey the relevant information to the public. The term "experimental," compared to the relevant circumstance of the vaccines we are talking about, appears technically correct and effective. What would be the alternative? In general, with respect to the short term and to the categories of people included in the initial studies, it can be probably said that the vaccines have already been tested and that we can therefore evaluate their risks and benefits (but I will return to this more specifically in the next chapter). Compared to the medium and long term, however, and to the categories of people not included in the initial studies, it can be safely said that the vaccines have not yet been tested and that they are therefore experimental, and that we do not know their effects and efficacy. On the other hand, how could something whose data for the experiment reside in the future have already been tested?

The surreptitious attempt by certain journalism (and certain TV experts) to recall alleged and improbable more technical meanings of the term "experimental" in order to mock the alleged (and mostly imaginary) anti-vaxxers is ridiculous and illogical. Language sometimes leads to linguistic conventions that are distant from the current spoken language. Philosophers know this well and are not in the least impressed. Therefore, admitted and not granted that, in some sectors of science today, the term "experimental" can conventionally mean something according to which the anti-Covid vaccines are no longer experimental (although we still have to wait to see what their use entails in the medium and long term and for certain categories of subjects: that is, although it is still necessary to *experience* them, in the meaning that this term has throughout the world from the 16th and 17th centuries onwards; that is, from the so-called scientific revolution forward), admitted and not granted, that is, that such a conventional use exists in some circles reserved for a few followers, this would not change anything with respect to the common meaning of the term and the substance of the information on anti-Covid vaccines to be communicated to the population.

There is a common semantic sense, perfectly reasonable and in accordance with the modern sense of the concept of *experimental science*, according to which current anti-Covid vaccines can and must be called "experimental." Those who do not understand this are stupid, in bad faith or blinded by some form of fanaticism.

4.7.1. Experimental Science and Predictivity

As I said, it is important to combine the concept of experimental science with that of predictivity that I have already mentioned.

Modern experimental science, in fact, links the experimental verification of scientific truths and/or hypotheses precisely to their predictive power. When a scientific truth is already tested, it assumes a precise predictive capacity on reality. The strength of experimental science lies precisely in the ability to predict the future. Construction science, for example, tells us with certainty that, if certain materials are used to build a flat roof, the roof will last for at least ten years, adequately performing its function of covering and protecting the building. Ten years is today the ordinary warranty term for flat roofs (at least in Italy), which means, for example, that if a roof causes infiltration problems before ten years from construction or renovation, save for the hypothesis of exceptional causes, the company that built it and the construction manager can be held accountable.

To understand the degree of experimentation and scientific strength of vaccines against Covid, we can use the same criterion and ask ourselves, for example, if the predictions on the efficacy of these vaccines and the achievement of herd immunity were well-founded. The answer, of course, is negative, and we have all become accustomed to the daily changing of indications and forecasts of vaccine efficacy and to the hypotheses of third, fourth, or perennial cyclic booster doses. This is not a polemical note but an epistemological one. Vaccine science is weak, and this weakness is a fact that has been *experimented* every day since these vaccines started being used. This weakness depends epistemologically on the fact that these vaccines have not yet been sufficiently tested, or *experimented*, to the point of acquiring the truth knowledge and predictive capacity of experimental science. Those who don't understand this know nothing interesting about experimental science and epistemology

4.7.2. The "Hoaxes" of the Italian National Institute of Health (ISS)

I want to give a concrete example of the disinformation and fanaticism that surrounds, at this moment, the epistemological aspects of the anti-Covid vaccine issue with reference above all to the theme of experimentation. The Italian Institute of Health (ISS) felt the need to create a handbook against hoaxes (bufale) and fake news circulating on these vaccines. The first of these hoaxes from which the ISS feels the need to urgently protect the population concerns precisely the issue we are discussing. Here it is:

> (Alleged) Hoax: "The short and long-term effects are unknown, the vaccines were produced too quickly and the only information comes from the companies."[58]

Faced with this alleged hoax, any intelligent person, even before reading the ISS refutation, makes an immediate logical analysis of the issue and asks:

a) Is this supposedly a single hoax or are they three different things?

b) Why are short-term effects combined with long-term ones?

c) Why is the speed aspect combined with that of information coming from companies?

The intelligent person immediately understands that there is something wrong because it is impossible to qualify that complex sentence as a single hoax but, above all, because it is made up of many small truths that are self-evident. Indeed::

a) It is certainly true that the long-term effects of vaccines are not known.

b) It is certainly true that the vaccines were produced quickly.

58 See Italian Institute of Health (ISS), "Covid: dall'Iss un vademecum contro le fake news sui vaccini", August 07, 2021, URL: https://www.iss.it/primo-piano/-/asset_publisher/3f4alMwzN1Z7/content/covid-dall-iss-un-vademecum-contro-le-fake-news-sui-vaccini.

c) It is certainly true that the information about the vaccines comes mostly from companies producing them.

It is the small tricks of those who wrote that sentence that generate one or more unlikely hoaxes:

a) Putting together "short and long term" is deceptive, because those who have doubts about these vaccines have them above all with respect to their long term side effects, while the short term effects are the only ones for which studies and clinical data already exist, albeit they are often limited;

b) "Too (quickly)" is per se questionable because it implies an unlikely evaluation judgment on what are the acceptable times for the production of vaccines;

c) "Only" obviously cannot be true because information on vaccines clearly comes (after authorization) from multiple sources.

The intelligent person immediately understands that here the hoax is that very sentence from the ISS and that the only reason to write such a senseless and deceptive sentence, presenting it as if it were a single hoax suggested by someone, is that the ISS needs to create a non-existent enemy to convey a certain message. Let's see, at this point, what the message is. Let's read the refutation of the alleged hoax against which the ISS intends to do justice.

“The pharmacovigilance system for SarsCov-2 vaccines is the same as for all other previously approved drugs and vaccines. After the results of the authorization studies carried out on tens of thousands of individuals of different ages, which were also conducted in this case, the reports from national and international regulatory agencies of possible adverse events temporally correlated with vaccination are collected. In case adverse events not manifested during the authorization studies are highlighted, if after a thorough investigation a causal relationship with vaccination is suspected or demonstrated, they are added to the list of adverse reactions, and which are listed in the information sheets of the various vaccines (pharmacovigilance post marketing)."[59]

Faced with this answer, the intelligent person literally leaps out of his skin. What does this answer have to do with the question? Where are the hoax and its refutation? In the face of the alleged hoax, the ISS does not clearly tell us whether the effects are known, or how quickly the vaccines were produced, or what information comes from companies and which information does not. Does it really make sense to present this type of information as if it were refuting a hoax? Isn't it rather the hoax that this type of information is provided by the ISS? Let's disprove the ISS hoax, then by analyzing the conceptual elements of this answer analytically. We can divide them into four:

a) Phaarmacovigilance system

Sure, the pharmacovigilance system is in itself the same as that used for other drugs and vaccines, but the phase that preceded the vaccine trade, in this case, and which depends only on the companies (with the control of the agencies), has been shortened and accelerated due to emergency. Therefore, these vaccines were put on the market very quickly— "too (quickly)", as I said, is an illogical evaluative term that ISS should not have used but which was used rhetorically for the creation of the false hoax—and with data from the companies alone. If we exclude the studies done only by companies for authorization purposes, the pharmacovigilance (third party) studies are triggered only after the vaccines have been placed on the market. It follows that this ISS statement on pharmacovigilance does not respond in any way to the surrepti-

59 Ibid.

tious questions put together in the alleged starting hoax. Pharmacovigilance does not imply that the short- and long-term effects are known, it does not imply that the vaccines have not been produced (too) quickly, and it does not imply that the (only) initial information does not come from companies. Question and answer are not logically and epistemologically linked here, except to a minimal and surreptitious degree.

b) Authorization studies

ISS cites authorization studies conducted on tens of thousands of individuals, but does not specify that these are initial studies made only by companies in conflict of interest and that they are still protected by trade secrets (nor does it mention the inherent limitations of these studies which I will return to in the next chapter). This information generates reliability in the naive reader due to the large number of people involved in the studies, but it is ambiguous since it surreptitiously avoids the initial question about the origin of the studies from the companies. Interestingly, almost all post-authorization studies, whether done by companies or independent, are done on very few people, even fewer than 100 per study. Some of these studies we will review in detail later. This is surprising if you think that after authorization it should be infinitely easier to have subjects on which to study the effects and efficacy of vaccines. How is it possible that before the authorization, it was possible to carry out studies so quickly on tens of thousands of people (willing to test a new drug on themselves) and then, when hundreds of millions of people are now using the vaccine and the entire independent scientific community can work on this, studies on a few hundred people can only be produced over a longer period of time? The only possible scientific hypothesis would seem to be that science strangely works better when it is carried out by companies alone with a view to authorization and remains secret.

c) Reports

The issue of the reports is cleverly inserted in the same period of the authorization studies ("After the results of the authorization...the reports...are collected") so that the unsuspecting reader does not even question the substantial difference between the two things. Naturally, the reports are a post-authorization event and therefore do not respond in any way to the questions of the alleged hoax. The reports, on the contrary: 1) logically imply that we do not already know all the effects of vaccines, certainly not the long-term ones, 2) say nothing about the exceptionally fast production of vaccines, and 3) say nothing about the origin of the vaccines' initial information. The reports only tell us that there will also be other sources of information on vaccines after they go on the market. How does this qualify the opening question as a hoax? At most, we could be faced with an explanation of the reporting system (which in this case is a crucial issue precisely because of the haste with which vaccines have been marketed, when there are so many unknowns about their efficacy and effects).

d) Post marketing pharmacovigilance

It is evident that the response of the ISS has nothing to do with those unlikely hoaxes created ad hoc. However, albeit in an ambiguous and deceptive context, it could have been at least an opportunity to clearly explain the difference between pre and post marketing pharmacovigilance. A wasted opportunity. The fact is that even this final reference does not answer the initial question and, frankly, I have never heard anyone question the post-authorization monitoring and updating of the leaflets, except for the way in

> which reports are collected on a voluntary basis, passively (and, often, with the difficult filter of health professionals who take the reports lightly, discouraging people to pursue them).

It is quite evident here that the ISS has invented a hoax (and in a somewhat clumsy way) just to make people believe, not what is written in its answer, but what is defined as a hoax in its question. In other words, the ISS's rhetorical goal was not to provide an adequate explanation of the pharmacovigilance or licensing studies mentioned in the answer (with respect to which it could have done much better), but to make people believe precisely that what is written in the clumsy description of the hoax is a hoax: that is, a) that the effects of vaccines are unknown, and b) that the vaccines were produced quickly c) on the basis of data coming solely from the pharmaceutical companies. Reading the ISS hoax page, people are led to think only about what's in the hoax description: that is, that these vaccines are exactly identical to any other drug or vaccine. The answer is indifferent; it must only provide a semblance of scientificity. This is a perfect example of misleading information.

Let's go to the second alleged hoax, which directly concerns the problem of vaccine testing (experimentation). Here it is, in the words of the ISS:

> (Alleged) Hoax: "Covid vaccines are experimental."[60]

To say that vaccines are experimental would therefore be the hoax. At least this alleged hoax, unlike the first, is expressed clearly and directly. Let's see how ISS explains this statement:

> "The term experimental vaccines (or drugs in general) refers to drugs not yet authorized for marketing. This is not the case with Covid-19 vaccines, the clinical use of which has been

60 Ibid.

> duly authorized by the EMA. In the case of COVID-19 vaccines, the development process has undergone an unprecedented acceleration globally. However, as the EMA itself reports on its website, *"a conditional authorization guarantees that the approved vaccine meets the strict EU criteria for safety, efficacy and quality, and that it is produced and controlled in approved and certified plants in line with pharmaceutical standards compatible with large-scale commercialization"*."[61]

The most obvious thing about this explanation is the change of discipline from medical science to law. The answer, in other words, is not based on a scientific meaning of what is experimental or not, nor on the meaning that ordinary language attributes to the scientific concept of being experimental. No, the explanation is based on a hypothetical legal criterion, according to which something is no longer experimental from the moment the authority decides to use it. That's like saying that if in the emergency of a war, it is decided to distribute machine guns to the soldiers while those guns are still in the testing phase, they become, at that precise moment, tested machine guns. What can I say? There are no alternatives here. Either whoever wrote these things is in bad faith and very clever, or he is in good faith but has, to say the least, an extremely limited logical capacity.

Let's assume that he is in good faith (which is an attitude that often leads to mistakes, but which makes us better) and let's distinguish between these two points of view ourselves, even if we lose some time doing so. As a lawyer, the idea that the law is stupid repels me. When an authority authorizes something for emergency reasons, it knows very well what it is doing and that there are risks. In other words, the law does not forget the substance of things; rather it tries to regulate everything as best as possible according to what it is. If something that is still being

61 Ibid.

tested is legally authorized, at the same time specific rules are envisaged to try to contain its unknowns and risks. It is the same legal concept of emergency or conditional authorization which, in the present case, embodies the scientific concept of a vaccine for which the testing process that science ordinarily requires has not been completed. All the specific rules related to emergency authorizations, including, for example, the follow-up obligations of pharmaceutical companies, the absence of alternatives or the effective reduction of hospitalizations, confirm the way in which the law recognizes and regulates the case of a vaccine authorized for use while it is still, at least to some extent, in an experimental phase. Not understanding this means having a somewhat grotesque idea of the law.

Therefore, even if we were to agree with the ISS that the adequate answer to the question on vaccine testing (or to the alleged hoax) should be placed at the legal level, we should respond that the ISS has totally misunderstood the meaning of the law and that it should instead pay attention to the meaning of the emergency legislation. Experimental is to science as emergency is to law. It is obvious, however, that we cannot agree with the ISS even on this approach, which we would only compliment by calling it reductive.

The concept of experimental concerns primarily and substantially the scientific plan and, in honest and correct communication, it must respect the substantial meaning that we all attribute to it. It is absurd to make fun of people about science by being pettifoggers with the law. The real hoax concerning vaccines is that of the ISS which states, on the basis of an irrelevant and misunderstood legal notion, that vaccines authorized in an emergency before the ordinary scientific process was completed, should be defined, not on the basis of science but on the basis of law, as already having been tested. It is also funny to read, in this surreal explanation, the reference to the unprecedented speed of the vaccine production process—a reference that was artfully avoided in the response to the first alleged hoax.

4.7.3. But Is There an Experimental Science of Adverse Effects?

At this point we must also clarify another aspect of the epistemology of the experimental science of anti-Covid vaccines (and drugs in general). The confusion of the current debate has in fact highlighted that too many people, starting with television experts, significantly confuse experimental science and the knowledge of adverse effects of vaccines/drugs.

So let's go back to the basic concept of experimental science, at least as we know it outside the twisted meanderings of entities such as the Italian ISS. Experimental science implies that the purely theoretical dimension of the sciences—at least of those sciences which imply the possibility of acting positively on the reality external to thought—cannot rise to a level of full and true reliability unless confirmed by a return, to put it this way, from theory to reality. *Mutatis mutandis*, it is a bit, at its level, like the *return to the phantasm* of which Thomas Aquinas speaks.[62] Sci-

62 In a nutshell, in Aquinas' Aristotelian thought, the abstract object of the intellect no longer has the same nature as reality. If the operation of the intellect stopped at abstraction, we would therefore have a split between thought and reality as the object of thought would be qualitatively and irreducibly different from actually existing things. In order for thought to be true and aligned with reality, it must therefore be able to see things as they really are by turning back to them the fruit of the operation of abstraction. This aspect of Thomist thought has often been expressed through the concept of intentionality, but I do not believe that this concept alone, without reflecting precisely on the return to phantasm and on the object proper to the intellect, can do justice to the depth of Aquinas' gnoseology. For Aquinas, the proper object of intellectual knowledge is not the universal as such (which is the object of second intention), but the essence of the really existing thing. I believe that the verifiability of the theory in experimental science is an application, albeit at a much less profound level, of the same gnoseological need that led Aquinas to the need to return to phantasm. See Thomas

(continued on the next page)

entific theory is in fact always an abstraction from reality (although often mediated by such a complex wealth of theoretical knowledge as to appear almost like a scientist's fantasy),[63] and abstraction is a process whose directionality proceeds from external reality towards thought. Science rises from theoretical to experimental when directionality is reversed, bringing theory back to the reality from which, by hypothesis, it arose. If the world is confirmed to function on the basis of theory, it can be said that it has been demonstrated and that the truth it expresses is now a truth that belongs no longer to theoretical science alone, but also to experimental science.

One of the most important aspects of experimental science is the replicability of the experiment. From this point of view, the vertex, or the definitive confirmation of the experimental truth, does not occur when some researchers successfully complete the experiment, but when other researchers, based on the same theoretical science and on the basis of the same parameters used for the experiment, are able to replicate it, confirming that in fact everything works as expected both theoretically and experimentally.

Repeatability is of course an aspect absent from the typical science of drugs because these are born, at the theoretical level, in a context of industrial secrecy, and even the clinical studies of the pre-authorization phase are shrouded in secrecy. The true scien-

---

Aquinas, *Summa theologiae*, I, q. 84, a. 7; F. Di Blasi, *God and the Natural Law*, sec. "2.2.2. The Object of Human Knowledge."

63 This is the reason why, at least from my point of view, authors like Thomas Samuel Kuhn can speak of scientific revolutions. See, e.g., Kuhn's well-known work *The Structure of Scientific Revolutions* (University of Chicago Press: Chicago, 1962). A serious scientific theory, however, even when it appears to be revolutionary or imaginative, is always the result of a theoretical thought qualified by years of study and experience by the scientist with his object of study. Scientific theory is never comparable to mere fantasy or science fiction.

tific community, therefore, is not effectively made aware of either the drug theory or the first experiments carried out using it.[64] The science of drugs, from this point of view (at least until the patents expire and trade secrets are no longer in force), does not respect adequate scientific parameters to be qualified as an experimental science.

Here, however, I want to focus on a more specific aspect, that of adverse effects. We already know that these effects are studied through epidemiology, which has a statistical nature. I have already said that statistics is a weak science and that it is not in itself capable of confirming a theory as it remains per se extraneous to why things happen the way they do. Let's pretend, however, that statistics are a valid tool for verifying theoretical science and ask ourselves what is the theoretical science of drugs that should be tested experimentally. After all, if a theoretical effect is expected and epidemiology then confirms it, it is possible, at least within certain parameters to be specified, to consider the statistical evidence as some kind of verification, albeit approximate, of the theoretical hypothesis.

But what does drug theory predict? In other words, if experimental science is that which verifies (*makes true* through facts) a theory, it is first necessary to confirm what the initial theoretical assumptions are. The underlying theory of the drug is the hypothesis of treating, preventing, or combating a certain disease with a certain degree of efficacy and safety. The theory of a particular drug, based on the principles and techniques used, can certainly imply the prediction of some adverse effects, and with respect to these expected effects one can see the epidemiology following the use of the drug (although, I repeat, in approximate

64 For some of these aspects and the FDA's resistance to administrative access to the records of the first full authorization of one of the anti-Covid vaccines (Pfizer's), I refer to my work, *The Death of the Phronimos: Faith and Truth about Anti-Covid Vaccines* (Phronesis editore: Palermo, 2021).

mode) as an experimental verification or as the experimental phase of drug science.

However, for the reasons I have already mentioned, almost none of the adverse effects of a new drug are predicted by the initial theory. The leaflets are mostly the result of subsequent additions of events never before anticipated. The epidemiology of post-authorization pharmacovigilance, from this point of view, is not experimental science, but a simple statistical survey with no scientific basis or explanations (which perhaps could theoretically be elaborated upon only after the detection of the problem). The relationship here is reversed. We don't have a theoretical science that is confirmed by experiments, and we don't even have experiments proper. We have statistics that detect events never predicted before and regarding which theoretical science begins to question itself after they occur (and as long as they are attributable to the drug).

When we talk about the experimental science of anti-Covid vaccines with respect to adverse effects, therefore, we use a scientifically very ambiguous language that attributes the certainty of experimental science to a field of knowledge that is in itself devoid of it. In the first authorization document of the first approved vaccine (Pfizer), for example, the section on known and unknown risks is almost non-existent and there is no theoretical mention of the adverse effects that began to characterize the discussion on vaccines in the months following its emergency authorization.[65] On the other hand, there have been theoretical hypotheses of adverse effects by independent scientists, based for example on the functioning of mRNA technologies and the Spike protein. The unusual thing is that these theoretical hypotheses were promptly rejected and ostracized by the public as if they were incompatible with the known science of vaccines, both

65 See FDA, Comirnaty and Pfizer-BioNTech COVID-19 Vaccine, "Decision Memorandum," December 11, 2020, URL: https://www.fda.gov/media/144416/download.

theoretical and experimental. But known by whom? Experimented how? Also from this point of view, the public debate that surrounded and surrounds anti-Covid vaccines is highly ambiguous and is clearly guided by interests and criteria external to true science.

4.8. Legal Immunity

Let's move now (but in a correct and not surreptitious way) from the scientific to the legal level. In fact, if we want to understand more fully the objective aspect of the circumstance on the medium and long term (and, in part, short term) unknown, we must focus on the legal immunity granted to pharmaceutical companies, physicians, and health professionals.

The story of this immunity begins long before Covid vaccines were put on the market. It begins in March 2020, in the study and production phase of these new products, when the United States of America decided to use the Public Readiness and Emergency Preparedness Act (PREP), a 2005 law that amended the Public Health Service Act (PHS), introducing the possibility of providing

> "liability immunity to certain individuals and entities (Covered Persons) against any claim of loss caused by, arising out of, relating to, or resulting from the manufacture, distribution, administration, or use of medical countermeasures (Covered Countermeasures), except for claims involving 'willful misconduct.'"[66]

66 See Federal Register, "Declaration Under the Public Readiness and Emergency Preparedness Act for Medical Countermeasures Against COVID-19," A Notice by the Health and Human Services Department on 03/17/2020, URL: https://www.federalregister.gov/documents/2020/03/17/2020-

(continued on the next page)

Thanks to The Pandemic and All-Hazards Preparedness Reauthorization Act (PAHPRA), 2013, the Covered Countermeasures of the PREP Act may include

> "products or technologies intended to enhance the use or effect of a drug, biological product, or device used against the pandemic or epidemic or against adverse events from these products."[67]

For the use of the PREP Act, the United States Secretary of Health and Human Services (what in other states is called the Minister of Health) had to both make a second health emergency declaration related to Covid—the first was on January 31, 2020, under the Public Health Service (PHS) Act—and define the activities, subjects, and limits of the immunity to be granted. The immunity provided by the Secretary of Health and Human Services has no geographical or population limits. The time limit should have been October 1, 2024, but the Secretary decided that an extension of 12 months was reasonable to accommodate the producers, which brought the deadline to October 2025. The subjects covered by immunity include manufacturers, distributors, program planners, qualified persons, and their officials, agents, and employees.

> "A manufacturer includes a contractor or subcontractor of a manufacturer; a supplier or licenser of any product, intellectual property, service, research tool or component or other article used in the design, development, clinical testing, investigation or manufacturing of a Covered Countermeasure; and any or all the parents, subsidiaries, affiliates, successors, and assigns of a manufacturer.
>
> A distributor means a person or entity engaged in the distribution of drugs, biologics, or devices, including but not

05484/declaration-under-the-public-readiness-and-emergency-preparedness-act-for-medical-countermeasures.

67 Ibid.

limited to: Manufacturers; re-packers; common carriers; contract carriers; air carriers; own-label distributors; private-label distributors; jobbers; brokers; warehouses and wholesale drug warehouses; independent wholesale drug traders; and retail pharmacies.

A program planner means a state or local government, including an Indian tribe; a person employed by the state or local government; or other person who supervises or administers a program with respect to the administration, dispensing, distribution, provision, or use of a Covered Countermeasure, including a person who establishes requirements, provides policy guidance, or supplies technical or scientific advice or assistance or provides a facility to administer or use a Covered Countermeasure in accordance with the Secretary's Declaration. Under this definition, a private sector employer or community group or other "person" can be a program planner when it carries out the described activities.

A qualified person means a licensed health professional or other individual authorized to prescribe, administer, or dispense Covered Countermeasures under the law of the state in which the Covered Countermeasure was prescribed, administered, or dispensed; or a person within a category of persons identified as qualified in the Secretary's Declaration. Under this definition, the Secretary can describe in the Declaration other qualified persons, such as volunteers, who are Covered Persons [...]

A person includes an individual, partnership, corporation, association, entity, or public or private corporation, including a federal, state, or local government agency or department."[68]

68 Ibid.

Indeed, this provides general immunity to anyone dealing with the new anti-Covid vaccines from the moment of their invention to the moment of vaccination.

4.8.1. Legal Negligence

It is quite evident that, in the face of an immunity clause so broad, generalized, and long-lasting, the very widespread idea touted by mainstream politics and journalism that these vaccines are like all the others and that, therefore, there is no reason to have fears or doubts about them, appears, to say the least, to be completely unfounded. If these vaccines were like all the others, those involved in their production and administration at any level would not need such unique and exceptional legal protection.

I repeat (as a jurist), here we are talking about an immunity provided for by emergency legislation which is in turn subject to a declaration of a national state of emergency. We are talking about an exception within an exception—anything but vaccines like all the others. From a legal and ethical point of view, people faced with the choice of using these vaccines should be informed both of the condition of emergency use authorization (EUA) and of the emergency legislation that underlies the legal immunity guaranteed to all citizens of the eccentric universe (outside the dimensions of science and law) in which these so-called vaccines exist.

Often we don't think enough about what this immunity means. Allow me, therefore, to dwell on it in different words, words like fault and negligence. Immunity means that we can be guilty of something but that we are not responsible for it to those who were harmed by our fault. It means that, in some areas of human action in which, due to their risks, specific rules or norms of conduct to follow are envisaged, we are exempt from liability for damage caused to third parties by our negligence: that is, by our culpable non-application or breach of these rules. It means escaping from any

> "liability claims alleging negligence by a manufacturer in creating a vaccine, or negligence by a health care provider in prescribing the wrong dose."[69]

Of course, many might think that immunity does not protect willful misconduct. There is a lot of naivety in this limit to immunity. Lawyers are well aware of how difficult it is to prove malice in a trial. Imagine facing hundreds of thousands of pages on tests and studies carried out on tens of thousands of people submitted by a pharmaceutical company to the FDA or EMA for marketing authorization. How can you prove that an error, even a significant one, in these studies and documents is the result of willful misconduct rather than culpable negligence? In fact, if there is no repentant witness, to do so would be almost impossible. In almost all court cases for damages or compensation, the concept that allows the verdict against the guilty party is that of fault, not that of willful misconduct. Adding willful misconduct to emergency legal immunity would be immoral and unthinkable both legally and politically, but not including it is, in fact, almost equivalent to including it.

Think now of the fabulous regime, the immense Christmas gift that this immunity generates for an industrial sector, such as the pharmaceutical one, famous for fraud and ethical indifference towards people's health and illness.[70] Pharmaceutical companies design and manufacture drugs in a regime of total autonomy and secrecy. The controls of the FDA or any other government agency are more theoretical than practical, also due to the inadequacy of resources and personnel of these bodies. Immunity adds to this autonomy and secrecy the security that any manipulation of data (done with sufficient care to avoid

69 Ibid.

70 I dwell on the history and curriculum of scandals and fraud in the pharmaceutical industry in my work, *The Death of the Phronimos: Faith and Truth about anti-Covid Vaccines*, op cit.

fraudulent evidence) will go unpunished. Even if, for example, gross errors were discovered on the risk-benefit assessment of a study, or on the identification of symptoms in clinical trial patients, or on the rupture of a double blind, or on the doses administered, or on the very number of patients involved and on the administration to them of the vaccine or placebo, all this would have no legal—civil or criminal—consequences.

What I want to emphasize here is not just that immunity is, as such, a circumstance that affects the relationship that an ethical subject must have with these vaccines. From this point of view, in fact, immunity is a sign of the uncertainty and objective danger of these new products, such that all those who work with them want to be guaranteed immunity. The general public can be made fun of and told not to worry, that these vaccines are just like all the others; but those who work with the vaccines are not fooled and want precise legal guarantees. This fact alone, however, only reveals, as I have already said, this: the objective danger of experimental drugs whose uncertainties do not make the experts calm. There is more, though.

Immunity makes vaccines less reliable because it facilitates data manipulation and negligence by everyone involved in the Covid vaccine assembly line—almost incentivizing these things, given the well-known cogs of the production and authorization of new drugs. Immunity will in fact statistically increase the attitude of pharmaceutical companies to overestimate all the positive things for their business and underestimate all the negative ones, especially in those pre-authorization phases in which companies can act in substantial autonomy and secrecy. Here, therefore, and above all, I want to emphasize that the existence of immunity enormously increases the level of prudent caution that one must have towards data on vaccines: data that come from pharmaceutical companies and that, precisely by virtue of the immunity these companies enjoy, will be less reliable and credible.

4.8.2. The Italian Criminal Shield (or Immunity)

There is no doubt that Europe has accepted various immunity clauses or limitations of liability for pharmaceutical companies in their famous sealed contracts (which even the European parliamentarians could not review freely). Furthermore, almost all European states have applied rules limiting civil and criminal liability for physicians and healthcare professionals. Here I will cite the Italian example, with which I am more familiar. In Italy, a so-called "criminal shield" has been provided for doctors and healthcare professionals who administer the vaccine.

In particular, a special provision of an exceptional nature has been included in this area by means of a government "decree law," which has immediate force of law, but which must subsequently be converted into ordinary law by Parliament. There was therefore an emergency process (that is, one that justifies the government's legislative initiative) which also involved the intervention of Parliament in a very short time. This norm was therefore considered particularly important by politics, to the point that it could not wait for an ordinary process. Let's read it:

> "Art. 3 (Criminal liability for administration of the anti SARS-CoV-2 vaccine)
>
> 1. For the facts referred to in articles 589 [manslaughter] and 590 [negligent personal injury] of the Criminal Code which occurred due to the administration of a vaccine for the prevention of SARS-CoV-2 infections, carried out during the extraordinary vaccination campaign in implementation of the plan referred to in article 1, paragraph 457, of law no. 178, PUNIBILITY IS EXCLUDED when the use of the vaccine complies with the indications contained in the marketing authorization provision issued by the competent authorities

> and with the circulars published on the institutional website of the Ministry of Health relating to vaccination activities."[71]

This rule, I repeat, approved urgently with the involvement of both the Government and the Parliament, perhaps reveals to the moral conscience that these vaccines are not like all the others more clearly than anything else could do. It must also be read in relation to the signature of *informed consent* that those who intend to receive the vaccine must provide. It is obvious, in fact, that it is very difficult for a doctor or a healthcare professional to incur criminal responsibility for the mere administration of a vaccine made according to the exceptional regulations in force. In this respect, no criminal shield would have been needed. Unless...

Unless they do something wrong in the prodromal activity to the administration. And what could they do in this prodromal phase that is so serious as to require a special criminal shield? Simple, they could give the wrong information on the risks and consequences of the vaccine, or they could review the patient's medical history superficially and end up recommending the vaccine lightly. In this case, the signature of the patient who acknowledges having been informed of all the pros and cons, of all the risks and of the anamnestic questionnaire, becomes essential precisely so that the health professionals can take advantage of the criminal shield.

> "It has been correctly observed that, in reality, the mere administration activity can hardly be the harbinger of culpable responsibility for death or injury of the vaccinated subject. Rather, it could be precisely the prodromal phase that concerns the compilation of a pre-vaccination triage form, an anamnestic questionnaire, and the collection of informed

71 Decree-Law April 1, 2021, n. 44, converted with amendments by Law May 28, 2021, n. 76 (in the Official Gazette May 31, 2021, n. 128). The underline and capital letters are mine.

consent on the possible adverse effects that the vaccine can cause following inoculation."[72]

Here we must reflect on the fact that a lot of information often given publicly by politicians and governments (and not without a rhetoric of false certainty as arrogant as it is superficial) would certainly imply serious civil and criminal liability if it were given by health professionals at the time of administering the vaccine. If a healthcare professional, using phrases pronounced by political authorities, said, for example, that getting vaccinated has no risk, that it is a civic duty, that everyone must do it, that the vaccine is 100% effective, that those who do not vaccinate themselves kill others, he or she would not be exempt from responsibility without the criminal shield.

Evidently, the criminal shield, in this context, serves to free from responsibility health professionals precisely in the event that they repeat to citizens at the time of vaccination the public lies told by the media and politicians about Covid vaccines, or in the event that, following the political line of the government,

---

72 See S. Marani, "L'esonero da responsabilità per la somministrazione di vaccino anti Covid-19," in *Altalex*, URL: https://www.altalex.com/documents/news/2021/07/06/esonero-da-responsabilita-per-somministrazione-vaccino-anti-covid-19). Mariani correctly takes up the interpretation of the criminal shield offered by the *Massimario della Cassazione*: see "Relazione n. 35 pubblicata 21/06/2021," *Ufficio del Massimario e del Ruolo della Corte di Cassazione*, URL: https://www.cortedicassazione.it/cassazione-resources/resources/cms/documents/Rel.35-2021.pdf. The *Corte di Cassazione* is the supreme court in Italy for disputes in civil and criminal matters. The *Massimario della Corte di Cassazione* is the office of the Court that deals with the systematic analysis of the decisions of the Court "conducted in order to create the conditions for useful and widespread information" regarding them: see Corte Suprema di Cassazione, "Massimario," URL: https://www.cortedicassazione.it/corte-di-cassazione/it/massimario.page.

they facilitate vaccination with superficial anamnesis. This criminal shield clearly serves to support the public legitimation of lies about vaccines operated by politics and aimed at pushing everyone to get vaccinated without ifs and buts. It should also be noted that the very existence of the criminal shield in Italy has not been publicized in the least by the authorities and the media, to the point that hardly anyone knows of its existence. As for other relevant issues, unfortunately, it has only been talked about a little in minor free-information media channels or alternative-news channels..

4.9. "Uncertainty about Risks": Epistemological Remarks

Let us now try to summarize the epistemological elements that emerged in this chapter with specific reference to this circumstance (internal institutional structural) of uncertainty about negative effects. Still, before doing so, let me remind you that this circumstance is identified, in this chapter, as a specific circumstance with reference only to the fact that the marketing of anti-Covid vaccines constituted an exception to the ordinary safety procedure of drug approval. There are other vaccine uncertainty profiles that relate to other more specific circumstances.

I also need to remind the readers that my attention to epistemological analysis is always functional to the ethical assessments of the circumstances. Therefore, I always try to summarize (at the cost of being repetitive) the truth aspects of the issues or factors that may affect ethical reasoning as linked to the one circumstance being dealt with each time. In other words, I am always interested in creating a functional link between the exposition of the epistemological findings and that of the ethical consequences. Sometimes, there is a direct correspondence between the two, in the sense that a specific epistemological consideration corresponds to a specific ethical evaluation. Other times, of course, this direct correspondence does not exist.

1) Experimental vaccines

To the extent that the anti-Covid vaccines have been put on the market before it was possible to fully observe and study their risks and consequences in the short, medium, or long term (in full or with respect to certain categories of people), they must be defined as experimental.

2) Science and predictive capacity

Experimental science implies predictive capacity. In the case of anti-Covid vaccines, a sign that they have not been approved on the basis of real experimental science already developed is that predictions about their efficacy and safety have not proved adequate and are constantly changing.

3) Not true experimental science

The main uncertainties that afflict people with regard to anti-Covid vaccines concern their adverse effects which, however, are not properly the subject of experimental science, but of mere statistical analysis to be carried out over a reasonably long time. Talking too much about experimental science regarding adverse effects is already a misleading way of providing information on drugs.

4) Institutional uncertainty

The legal framework surrounding anti-Covid vaccines attests to the uncertainty about their risks in various ways. This uncertainty is therefore a structural or institutional part of truth talk about these products.

5) Truth of the law

The law (contracts, immunities, criminal shield, etc.), as it implies responsibility, brings out the shareable and reliable truths of the issues it regulates. This makes it an excellent epistemological reference point for evaluating what people, private entities and institutions are certain about and what they are not.

6) Cognitive gamble

In the case of anti-Covid vaccines, we cannot properly speak of risk-benefit assessment. Evaluating the risks and benefits means comparing them, but a comparison presupposes knowledge of the terms of the comparison. In this case, some of the terms are unknown and therefore cannot logically be compared with the known ones. The relevant operation, therefore, looks more like a bet or gamble and must be analyzed epistemologically as such.

7) Leaflets

With regard to leaflets, the logical difference between anti-Covid vaccines and other regularly approved drugs or vaccines is that, in the case of the former, leaflets do not exist. There are only information sheets that are constantly updated which cannot offer any guidance regarding unknown risks, especially those over the medium and long term.

8) Guesswork

It is possible to make professional decisions in areas where data is lacking or there is insufficient data. In these cases, one operates through intuition or conjecture. Decisions made in this way have a more or less high degree of uncertainty and unpredictability but are not irrational. The important thing is that the part or portion of the decision based on intuition is adequately identified (for example, 20% of the relevant decision relating to the missing data X) and that it is adequately argued in itself and with respect to the overall decision. The decision is rational, even if partially uncertain and unpredictable, to the exact extent in which the points to be left to guesswork are identified and adequately argued. The guesswork of the government agencies responsible for Covid vaccines concerning unknown future risks does not seem to be identified and argued in an epistemologically correct and exhaustive way.

9) Weakness of statistics

The epidemiological studies with which the risks and negative effects of drugs and vaccines are ascertained are mainly statistical. Statistics is a weak truth knowledge that has many margins of error in the selection of data, in data collection, and in the development of adequate and complete mathematical models.

10) Limits of statistics

Statistics cannot express any truth, albeit weak, on data that it has not yet elaborated. The unknown future risks of vaccines cannot be the object of epidemiological truths until they pass from the present to the past, becoming known and part of the acquired data.

4.10. "Uncertainty about Risks": Ethical Consequences

Let us now summarize, also in function of the epistemological findings highlighted, and with respect to the specific circumstance of the objective uncertainty of the negative effects, the ethical consequences of this circumstance for the moral conscience. Summarizing these consequences serves to highlight the importance that the circumstance in question can assume in the ethical reasoning of the person who reflects on these vaccines in order to decide what to do about them. Remember that these conceptual summaries are purely illustrative and in no way exhaustive. Let me also remind the reader that it is not good to make ethical decisions based on a single circumstance (unless it is exclusionary) and/or on a single ethical consideration (unless it concerns an exclusionary circumstance).

1) Strong intrinsic doubt

   The uncertainty about the risks due to the hasty and/or emergency authorizations of anti-Covid vaccines generates in itself a strong intrinsic doubt with regard to the possible choice to use them. Unknown risks are not something to be taken lightly and require a bet based on significant, certain, and evident advantages.

2) Non-exclusionary circumstance

   This circumstance cannot be understood in any way as exclusionary, in the sense that it does not necessarily indicate that the choice of the vaccine is wrong or that it is wrong in some cases. At the level of architectural or systematic analysis of the circumstance in question, it is only required that the moral agent takes it into consideration with due attention.

3) Right to information

   The relevance of this circumstance implies the right to be adequately informed by the authorities and health professionals in order to be able to make one's own free evaluation in this regard.

4) Bet or gamble

It is essential that the agent understands that the risk-benefit assessment, in this case, is not a true assessment—as it would be in cases where you know exactly what the risks and what the benefits are. The leaflets do not exist; even if one wanted to read them, he could not do it. The choice implies a leap in the dark, a gamble, which can be more or less dangerous according to the other circumstances to be evaluated in the specific case. The jump (or bet), for example, is very different in the cases of a 12-year-old child and of a 75-year-old adult.

5) No institutional certainties

The moral agent must know that political and scientific authorities do not have strong certainties, as emerges unequivocally from official documents and regulations (even if not from public information).

6) False certainties

The moral agent must reflect on the fact that any certainties displayed by people in the mass media are a scam or, in very few cases, a mistake made in good faith by ignorant people.

7) Experimental vaccines

The moral agent must know that vaccines are experimental (i.e., in their testing phase) with respect to the medium and long term both as to their efficacy and, and above all, as to their potential negative effects. Anti-Covid vaccines are partly experimental even with respect to the short term, which is why all forecasts on the timing and effectiveness of vaccine protection have not worked. Experimental science does not fail in comparison with facts because it is the comparison with facts that previously established it as a scientific knowledge. If the predictions of vaccines have failed even in the medium term, this is proof that these products had not been tested or that they had been tested by means of a mediocre and fallacious science. He who uses these vaccines must know that he is taking part in a trial, or experimenting with the vaccines, in whole or in part, on himself.

8) Consent to experimentation

What has just been said naturally affects the consent to the use of these "vaccines" because this consent must be explicitly given in relation to the acceptance of an experimental therapy on oneself.

9) Weaks truths about vaccines

Statistical or epidemiological truths about the risks or effectiveness of anti-Covid vaccines, even when correctly processed on existing data, should never be presented on a par with strong or absolutely certain scientific truths. A reasonable doubt must be expressed towards those who present them in this way without making the appropriate clarifications. The repeated failures of forecasts on efficacy, herd immunity, or number of doses needed highlight the unreliability of current vaccine science, which often should not be presented in terms of "science" without the appropriate qualifications

10) Immunity and criminal shield

The various immunities that characterize the universe of current anti-Covid vaccines have a double ethical value. On the one hand, they reveal per se the uncertainty surrounding the risks and benefits of these products. On the other hand, they create a favorable context for manipulation of data and/or for dishonesty and negligence in the use of data by pharmaceutical companies. Immunity both raises doubts and damages pre-authorization research on vaccines.

Chapter 5

Emergency and Conditional Authorizations

The lack of certainty about negative effects has meant that the anti-Covid vaccines were gradually authorized on the market by the appropriate agencies (FDA for the United States and EMA for Europe)[73] on the basis of emergency authorizations—or conditioned authorizations, as they are called in Europe—due to the absence of the availability of other drugs or therapies. Let's read what these authorizations mean from the same agencies in charge of Europe and the United States.

U.S. Food and Drug Administration:

> "Emergency Use Authorization for Vaccines Explained: An Emergency Use Authorization (EUA) is a mechanism to facilitate the availability and use of medical countermeasures, including vaccines, during public health emergencies, such as the current COVID-19 pandemic. Under an EUA, FDA may allow the use of unapproved medical products, or unapproved uses of approved medical products in an emergency to diagnose, treat, or prevent serious or life-

73 Technically, the EMA recommends approval which is then decided by the European Commission.

threatening diseases or conditions when certain statutory criteria have been met, including that there are no adequate, approved, and available alternatives."[74]

European Medicines Agency (EMA):

"Conditional marketing authorisation:
The approval of a medicine that addresses unmet medical needs of patients on the basis of less comprehensive data than normally required. The available data must indicate that the medicine's benefits outweigh its risks and the applicant should be in a position to provide the comprehensive clinical data in the future."[75]

The possibility of emergency authorization for the use of drugs (EUA) is provided and governed, in the U.S. system, by section 564 of a federal law, the *Federal Food, Drug, and Cosmetic Act* (FD&C Act). That section was incorporated into this law by the *Project Bioshield Act* of 2004, which is a law aimed at amending

> "the Public Health Service Act to provide protections and countermeasures against chemical, radiological, or nuclear

74 See FDA, "Emergency Use Authorization for Vaccines Explained," URL: https://www.fda.gov/vaccines-blood-biologics/vaccines/emergency-use-authorization-vaccines-explained.

75 See *European Medicines Agency* (EMA), "Conditional marketing authorization," URL: https://www.ema.europa.eu/en/glossary/conditional-marketing-authorisation. There are currently five vaccines with conditional authorization in Europe by the EMA, each with specific clinical data, potential side effects and clinical tests: see "COVID-19 vaccines: authorized," https://www.ema.europa.eu/en/human-regulatory/overview/public-health-threats/coronavirus-disease-covid-19/treatments-vaccines/vaccines-covid-19/covid-19-vaccines-authorised#authorised-covid-19-vaccines-section.

> agents that may be used in a terrorist attack against the United States by giving the National Institutes of Health contracting flexibility, infrastructure improvements, and expediting the scientific peer review process, and streamlining the Food and Drug Administration approval process of countermeasures."[76]

These rules are therefore inserted in the context of the U.S. national defense system against terrorist attacks of a biological or chemical nature (such as the anthrax attacks in 2001), also allowing the accumulation and possible emergency use of vaccines that have not yet been tested on human beings. The exception to drug safety for reasons of national emergency is inherent in this legislation and has always been its most delicate ethical aspect.

Let me recall that the institutes mentioned in this introduction to the law—the National Institutes of Health and the Food and Drug Administration (FDA), but also the CDC—are all part of the United States Department of Health and Human Services (HHS), which is equivalent to what in other states would be called the federal government's health ministry. It is therefore normal for the law to focus on the special powers conferred, in relevant matters, on the minister or head of the department: i.e., the Secretary of Health and Human Services. It is the Secretary of Health, for example, who declares a state of health emergency. All decisions on emergency authorizations are either up to him or fall under his jurisdiction or sphere of competence.

The first declaration of a state of emergency, the one that preceded and allowed the EUAs, dates back to January 2020 and is clearly motivated by the evolution of a dangerous situation

76 See U.S.A. "*Project Bioshield Act of 2004,*" URL: https://www.congress.gov/108/plaws/publ276/PLAW-108publ276.pdf.

in American territory. Indeed, it would be ethically unacceptable to require citizens of a state to limit their fundamental rights and subject them to experimental health treatment if the emergency risk were theoretical or too distant from them to pose a real threat. The effectiveness of emergency and security measures requires the immediacy of the threat or risk. A proportion is needed between the proximity and effectiveness of the emergency danger, on the one hand, and the infringement of rights and the approval of experimental therapies on the other.

> "As a result of confirmed cases of 2019 Novel Coronavirus (2019-nCoV), on this date and after consultation with public health officials as necessary, I, Alex M. Azar II, Secretary of Health and Human Services, pursuant to the authority vested in me under section 319 of the Public Health Service Act, do hereby determine that a public health emergency exists and has existed since January 27, 2020, nationwide."[77]

As for Europe,

> "EMA's CHMP [*Committee for Medicinal Products for Human Use*] may grant a conditional marketing authorisation for a medicine if it finds that all of the following **criteria** are met:
>
> - the benefit-risk balance of the medicine is positive;
> - it is likely that the applicant will be able to provide comprehensive data post-authorisation;
> - the medicine fulfils an unmet medical need;

77 See U.S.A. *Secretary of Health and Human Services*, "Determination that a Public Health Emergency Exists," January 31, 2020, URL: https://www.phe.gov/emergency/news/healthactions/phe/Pages/2019-nCoV.aspx.

- the benefit of the medicine's immediate availability to patients is greater than the risk inherent in the fact that additional data are still required."[78]

Conditional authorization is governed in Europe by Regulation no. 507 of 2006.[79] This document is in perfect conceptual harmony with the American emergency authorization regulations. It clarifies, for example, that the scope concerns the "treatment, prevention or diagnosis of seriously disabling or life-threatening diseases," the "medicines to be used in emergency situations in response to threats to public health," or the so-called "orphan drugs."[80]

5.1. Specific Presuppositions of Emergency Authorizations

Even from these brief general regulatory notes, the key criteria or presuppositions of these authorizations emerge immediately. Let's summarize them briefly, combining both FDA and EMA's

78 Cfr., *European Medicines Agency* (EMA), Conditional marketing authorisation, URL: https://www.ema.europa.eu/en/human-regulatory/marketing-authorisation/conditional-marketing-authorisation#use-during-covid-19-pandemic-section.

79 See Regulation (EC) no. 507/2006 of the Commission of March 29, 2006 relating to the conditional marketing authorization of medicinal products for human use that fall within the scope of Regulation (CE) no. 726/2004 of the European Parliament and of the Council: URL: https://eur-lex.europa.eu/eli/reg/2006/507/oj.

80 See ibid. art 2. Orphan medicines concern particularly serious pathologies for which valid treatment systems do not exist. They are defined in art. 3 of Regulation (EC) no. 141/2000 of the European Parliament and of the Council of December 16, 1999: URL: https://eur-lex.europa.eu/legal-content/EN/TXT/?uri=CELEX%3A32000R0141.

principles because the ethical profile that interests me at the moment has no territorial or legal-positivist boundaries.

1) Health emergency

    Existence of a medical emergency or a state of emergency, which must be officially declared by a competent government authority.

2) Lack of alternatives

    Lack of alternatives to deal with the medical emergency. That is, "that there is no adequate, approved, and available alternative to the product for diagnosing, preventing, or treating such disease or condition" (FD&C Act, sec. 564).

3) Threat

    Threat represented by a fatal disease, which the FDA calls "serious or life-threatening disease" and which the EMA, more prosaically (but in line with Article 4 of Regulation 507/2006), calls an "unmet medical need".

4) Guarantee of efficacy

    Guarantee of efficacy, which is an implicit requirement in the entire emergency legislation since the drug must provide a benefit or positive contribution to the solution of the emergency: it must fight the disease, meet the unmet medical need, etc.

a. Reduction of hospitalizations

    This is an implicit requirement with respect to the efficacy of the authorized product: that is, its ability to cope with the national health emergency. If, in the face of a health emergency that clogs hospitals, the product approved in emergency mode does not create an appreciable reduction in hospitalizations, it means that it does not work and that the authorization is not justified by the efficacy of the product.

5) Benefit-risk ratio

This requirement has several important aspects that deserve specific analysis, including:

a. Positivity

It must be positive in general, in the sense that the benefits must always outweigh the risks.[81]

b. Clear assessment methods

It must explain the methods of assessing future and unknown risks.

c. Monitoring

It must provide effective and adequate methods for monitoring these risks.

d. Assistance in case of adverse effects

81 "The known and potential benefits of the product, when used to diagnose, prevent, or treat such disease or condition, outweigh the known and potential risks of the product": see Project Bioshield Act 2004, amending the Federal Food, Drug, and Cosmetic Act by inserting the EUA legislation in section 564, URL: https://www.congress.gov/108/plaws/publ276/PLAW-108publ276.pdf.

It must provide for special and adequate methods of assistance for people who may suffer negative consequences from the use of the drug. These people not only cannot be abandoned, but must be helped in a preferential and superlative way as they are part of a medical experiment for the common good.

e. Positive balance between immediacy and risks

It must offer a positive balance between the immediacy of the measure and the missing scientific data, in the sense that the advantage of the immediate availability of the drug must be more important than the risks deriving from incomplete scientific data.

f. Confirmation at the end of the experiment

Its evaluation must be confirmed after authorization in light of the completion of studies and trials on the drug.[82]

6) Obligation to provide complete data

Availability and ability of manufacturers to provide missing or incomplete drug data in the future. This, of course, is a requirement that logically follows the fact that emergency approval causes a product that is still under study and testing to be placed on the market.

82 See Regulation (EC) no. 507/2006, op. cit., art. 5: "The holder of a conditional marketing authorization has a specific obligation to complete ongoing studies or to conduct new studies in order to confirm that the benefit / risk balance is positive and to provide additional data [...]." The emphasis is mine.

7) More pharmacovigilance

A strengthening of pharmacovigilance given that, in fact, the nature of the emergency authorizations brings with it greater risks for those who will take the drugs.
"Enhanced pharmacovigilance for medicinal products granted a conditional marketing authorisation is important and is already adequately provided for in Directive 2001/83/EC and Regulation (EC) No 726/2004."[83]

Each of these aspects would deserve a separate discussion as it is suitable, even on its own, to determine the ethical choice on individual products both by the competent authorities and by individual patients or citizens faced with the possibility of administering the experimental drug. Some of the issues involved in the analysis of these aspects are absolutely crucial. I will provide three examples, one on the risk-benefit assessment, one on the lack of alternatives, and one on efficacy.

5.1.1. Assessment According to Stakeholder Groups

One thing that has been talked about too little is that the risk-benefit assessment should be done in relation to each population group that has different relationships with the disease and the vaccine. Some groups of subjects, such as pregnant women, those who have recovered from Covid, various subjects with comorbidities and the immunocompromised, as I have already pointed out on other occasions, were not even included in the initial pre-authorization studies. With regard to those subjects, therefore,

83 See ibid. point "(11)".

the risk-benefit ratio was logically unjustified with respect to existing scientific data, and it was illegitimate and immoral to allow them to be administered experimental drugs following an authorization that clearly did not concern them, not having taken them into consideration.

In the meeting of the FDA Advisory Committee of 10 June 2021, concerning the possible extension of the EUA to pediatric groups from 6 months to 18 years, the FDA officer in charge of reporting on the emergency regulation talked about this aspect in specific reference to the age factor:

> "[...] statutory criteria for EUA [...] sufficient data to support that the vaccine's known and potential benefits outweigh known and potential risks in the age group(s) being considered for EUA."[84]

In this regard, it is of utmost importance to have a serious and open scientific discussion on the way in which groups of subjects for which the risk-benefit ratio could not be evaluated with specific scientific data were actually included in the emergency authorizations, or for which there could not be a logical link between the data available and the conclusions outlined in the EUA provision. The lack of adequacy between premises and conclusions is a very serious logical error in administrative measures that involve people's health and lives.

5.1.2. Lack of Alternatives?

In the summary document of the criteria of Pfizer's first emergency authorization, the FDA expressed in these terms the requirement of the lack of alternatives:

> "No vaccine or other medical product is FDA approved for prevention of COVID-19 [...] Thus, there is

84 See FDA, "Advisory Committee meeting 10/06/2021," D. Fink, presentation slide at 2:32:21, URL: https://www.youtube.com/watch?v=70Xhn3K9SlQ&t=14915s.

> currently no adequate, approved, and available alternative for prevention of COVID-19."[85]

A jurist here immediately notices a discrepancy between the general requirement that "there is currently no adequate, approved, and available alternative"—and that there is "an unmet medical need" (EMA)—and the detailed application of it that the FDA makes, saying that "No vaccine or other medical product is FDA approved for prevention of COVID-19."

Indeed, here it seems that by alternative available or unmet medical need we only restrictively mean the existence of a specific drug approved by the FDA for Covid-19. The application to the specific case, in other words, is clearly more restrictive than the general criterion and, for example, is not suitable for including, among the available alternatives, non-drug therapies, social prevention rules, vitamins, or off-label uses of other drugs.

To be critical, it could be said that this judgment was structured specifically to exclude from the evaluation of the available alternatives, for example, early therapies, the off-label use of traditional drugs, and the medical profession in general, all intended to care for the patient by stimulating the natural reaction of the immune system and not just to prescribe drugs as approved by an agency.

The decision in favor of Pfizer that I have just referenced seems to be the result of an unbalanced conceptual clash between real medicine—the one that cannot function without including the relationship between the doctor and his patient—and an abstract or disembodied medicine reduced to institutional pharmacology, in which the doctor is only a bureaucratized intermediary between the drug agency and the patient. But is medicine the science of FDA approved drugs, or is it something more and different?

---

85 See FDA, Comirnaty and Pfizer-BioNTech COVID-19 Vaccine, "Decision Memorandum," December 11, 2020, URL: https://www.fda.gov/media/144416/download.

5.1.3. Efficacy of Vaccines?

The requirement of efficacy has become very problematic due also to the failure of any forecast in this regard. For, as I will explain shortly, it is one of those requirements that raises the greatest problems of conflicts of interest and diachronic evaluations. The official news on the efficacy of the Pfizer vaccine, for example, was particularly erratic in the days before and after the final authorization of the FDA. Indeed, for the authorization, a strong efficacy was needed and so it was presented. After approval, however, a waning efficacy was needed in order to launch the third dose market, and so it was presented. Out of the blue, the efficacy was significantly reduced, but this did not in the least lead to any questioning of the (political) authorization that had just been granted to the vaccine. I will return to this later.

Here I want to recall a topic related to the efficacy of vaccines that has not been talked about much. And I want to do it just to give an idea of how broad and varied a serious and scientific discussion on this requirement must be.

5.1.3.1. They Had Not Been Tested for their Touted Efficacy

Some scholars have expressed doubts that the discussion on efficacy during the authorization phase focused above all on the development of symptoms of the disease. Many people, in fact, do not reflect enough on the difference between the SARS-CoV-2 virus (acronym for: severe acute respiratory syndrome coronavirus 2) and Covid 19 disease. The two are different in nature. But does the vaccine that is approved or to be approved have to be effective against the virus or against the disease? Does it have to make people immune and stop contagions, or does it have to alleviate the symptoms and effects of the disease?

It is now increasingly evident that these vaccines are not effective with respect to infections and therefore do not grant immunity from the virus, but the fact is that they had never been tested to evaluate their effectiveness on the virus. This is perhaps the reason (or one of the reasons) why the CDC, as we will see, felt the need to change the definition of a vaccine, which traditionally has always focused on conferring immunity and not on alleviating symptoms. If a vaccine is just a drug that relieves symptoms, then aspirin is a vaccine.

It is also not true, however, contrary to what the general public has been led to believe, that the vaccines approved in an emergency way give guarantees to avoid the serious consequences of the disease in terms of hospitalizations and deaths. Pre-authorization studies weren't even designed to give these kinds of results. This is another example of an ethically unacceptable discrepancy between reality and what was communicated to the public.[86]

It is the chief medical officer at Moderna—Peter Doshi tells us—who admits this. The serious adverse effects of Covid are too rare to be observed in a group of people of even thirty or forty thousand participants. Furthermore, the elderly popula-

86 "Peter Hotez, dean of the National School of Tropical Medicine at Baylor College of Medicine in Houston, said, "Ideally, you want an antiviral vaccine to do two things . . . first, reduce the likelihood you will get severely ill and go to the hospital, and two, prevent infection and therefore interrupt disease transmission." Yet the current phase III trials are not actually set up to prove either. None of the trials currently under way are designed to detect a reduction in any serious outcome such as hospital admissions, use of intensive care, or deaths. Nor are the vaccines being studied to determine whether they can interrupt transmission of the virus" (P. Doshi, "Will Covid-19 Vaccines Save Lives? Current Trials Aren't Designed to Tell Us," *BMJ*, Published October 21, 2020, 371:m4037, doi:10.1136/bmj.m4037). See also P. Doshi, D. Light, "How to Expand Access to COVID Vaccines without Compromising the Science. Emergency use authorizations by the FDA are not ideal," *Scientific American*, December 17, 2020, URL: https://www.scientificamerican.com/article/how-to-expand-access-to-covid-vaccines-without-compromising-the-science/.

tion, which is the most affected by this type of event, was not sufficiently represented in the trials to give any relevant results.

> "But Tal Zaks, chief medical officer at Moderna, told *The BMJ* that the company's trial lacks adequate statistical power to assess those outcomes. "The trial is precluded from judging [hospital admissions], based on what is a reasonable size and duration to serve the public good here," he said. Hospital admissions and deaths from Covid-19 are simply too uncommon in the population being studied for an effective vaccine to demonstrate statistically significant differences in a trial of 30,000 people. The same is true of its ability to save lives or prevent transmission: the trials are not designed to find out. Zaks said, "Would I like to know that this prevents mortality? Sure, because I believe it does. I just don't think it's feasible within the timeframe [of the trial] [...] "Our trial will not demonstrate prevention of transmission," Zaks said, "because in order to do that you have to swab people twice a week for very long periods, and that becomes operationally untenable"."[87]

Despite what the population has been led to believe by political communications and the mainstream mass media, the data on the effectiveness of the pre-authorization studies are based on weak statistics[88] and on very few final actual numbers drawn from one hundred or two hundred people.[89]

---

87 Ibid.

88 "Moderna, like Pfizer and Janssen, has designed its study to detect a relative risk reduction of at least 30% in participants developing laboratory confirmed covid-19" (ibid).

89 "Covid-19 vaccine trials are currently designed to tabulate final efficacy results once 150 to 160 trial participants develop symptomatic covid-19—and most trials have specified at least one interim analysis allowing for the trials to end with even fewer data accrued. Medscape's Eric Topol has been a vocal critic of the trials' many interim analyses. "These numbers seem totally out of line with what would be considered

(continued on the next page)

5.1.3.2. Pfizer Data and Report 9

Let me try to explain this aspect a little better to make it more understandable and concrete. To this end, I move from Moderna to Pfizer which, among the various vaccines, is the one that has used the largest number of volunteers in the relevant clinical trials. For the purposes of Pfizer's emergency authorization, data from the—phases 1/2/3—study C4591001 were used. Phases 2 and 3 of this study involved 43,448 people, of whom 21,720 received the vaccine and 21,728 received a placebo. The average age of the participants was 51 .[90]

Let's now take a step back to Report 9, the famous document drawn up after the first months of the pandemic (the hardest even in terms of mortality), which—given that any vaccines would not have been available, according to the most optimistic scientific forecasts, before "potentially 18 months or more"—offered an analysis of non-pharmacological tools that governments could have used in the meantime (protection of those most at risk, quarantines, social distancing, etc.). Report 9 was at that time a crucial document in the world to evaluate the immediate political reactions for containment of the pandemic.[91]

---

stopping rules," he says. "I mean, you're talking about giving a vaccine with any of these programs to tens of millions of people. And you're going to base that on 100 events?" (ibid).

90 See FDA, "Vaccines and Related Biological Products Advisory Committee Meeting December 10, 2020 - FDA Briefing Document, Pfizer-BioNTech COVID-19 Vaccine," URL: https://www.fda.gov/media/144245/download#page=46. Of course, study C4591001 is still ongoing and will end in 2023. I refer here to the partial data used in December 2020 for the emergency authorization.

91 N. Ferguson, D. Faydon, G. Nedjati Gilani, N. Imai, K. Ainslie, M. Baguelin, S. Bhatia, A. Boonyasiri, Z. Cucunuba Perez, G. Cuomo-Dannenburg, A. Dighe, I. Dorigatti, H. Fu, K. Gaythorpe, W. Green, A. Hamlet, W. Hinsley, L. Okell, S. Van Elsland, H. Thompson, R. Verity, E. Volz, H. Wang, Y. Wang, P. Walker, C. Walters, P. Winskill,

(continued on the next page)

Table 1 of Report 9 offers "current estimates" of Covid 19 cases divided by hospitalization, intensive care, and death. Of course, the figures increase exponentially over the age of 70, reaching over age 80 to 70.9% intensive care and 9.3% death. However, if we consider the bands related to the average age of the Pfizer C4591001 study, things change enormously. Intensive care is on average at 5%, while deaths are almost non-existent. Here are the exact figures cited:

Table 1: Current estimates of the severity of cases

Age-group (years)	% symptomatic cases requiring hospitalisa-tion	% hospitalised cases requiring critical care	Infection Fata-lity Ratio
0-9	0.1%	5.0%	0,002%
10-19	0.3%	5.0%	0,006%
20-29	1.2%	5.0%	0,03%
30-39	3.2%	5.0%	0,08%
40-49	4.9%	6.3%	0,15%
50-59	10.2%	12.2%	0,60%
60 to 69	16.6%	27.4%	2.2%
70 to 79	24.3%	43.2%	5.1%
80+	27.3%	70.9%	9.3%

The 50-59 range, of course, is already far beyond the average age of the Pfizer study. What do these numbers mean?

C. Whittaker, C. Donnelly, S. Riley, A. Ghani, "Report 9: Impact of non-pharmaceutical interventions (NPIs) to reduce COVID19 mortality and healthcare demand," *Imperial College COVID-19 Response Team* , March 16, 2020, Published Online, URL: https://spiral.imperial.ac.uk/handle/10044/1/77482.

They mean that out of a population of 100,000 people, the expected mortality from Covid will be 2 people for the 0-9 age range, 6 for the 10-19 age group, 30 for the 20-29 age group, etc., up to the highest band under 50 where the expected mortality would be 150 people. However, Pfizer's study only used 43,448 people, so we need to more than halve those numbers. The people involved in Pfizer's study seem to be many in themselves, but compared to the "death from Covid" event, they are a statistically insignificant number. This already gives a more precise idea of Tal Zaks' conclusion reported above.

Still, let's now review some of the actual data from study C4591001 to get an even more adequate idea of the problem. Of course, my goal here is not to provide any kind of general interpretation of the relevant study, but only to give the reader an idea of the reference numbers for evaluation purposes.

To evaluate the efficacy of the vaccine, the participants were monitored after vaccination for at least seven days.[92] The average follow-up for all participants was two months. The first cut-off date was November 4, 2020, "when a total of 94 confirmed COVID-19 cases were accrued." At the cut-off date of November 14, 2020, "a total of 170 confirmed COVID-19 cases were accrued." When we shift the goal from the high-sounding numbers of 44,000 people to the modest numbers of 170 Covid cases, the perspective from which to evaluate the results of the studies changes considerably. For example, let's shift our focus to the overall results of deaths and adverse effects indicated as reasons for the withdrawal from the study. This is an excerpt from

92 "All of the participants included in the first interim efficacy analysis had at least 7 days of follow-up after Dose 2, and thus were enrolled no later than October 7, 2020" (FDA, "Vaccines and Related Biological Products Advisory Committee Meeting December 10, 2020 - FDA Briefing Document, Pfizer-BioNTech COVID-19 Vaccine," op. cit.).

Table 3 of the Analysis Document used by the FDA Vaccine Evaluation Committee:[93]

Table 3. Disposition of All Randomized Participants, Phase 2/3 Safety Population

Treatment Group	BNT162b 2 N=18904 n (%)	Placebo N=18892) n (%)	Total N=37796 n (%)
Reason for Withdrawal:			
- **Adverse Event**	8 (0.0)	5 (0.0)	13 (0.0)
- **Death**	2 (0.0)	4 (0.0)	6 (0.0)

You will notice easily that here all percentages are shown in 0.0 because 2, 4 or 6 cases out of 18,904, 18,892 or 37,796 respectively represent less than 0.0 percent. These numbers both in absolute terms and in percentage terms are clearly irrelevant with respect to the study carried out. They are obviously unable to provide any appreciable results. Apart from the case of death, the adverse events in this table are interesting to me because they were reasons for the withdrawal of people (still living) from the study. Now of course I don't know what happened in the specific withdrawal cases, but I hypothesize that people who had really serious adverse events had to be cured by breaking the double blind. Who would remain in a blind trial at risk of dying? It therefore seems reasonable to me that the most serious adverse events are among the reasons for the withdrawal. If this is true, it also means that the efficacy results of the drug could not include serious adverse events due to both the statistically insignificant number of the same and because these events led to the with-

93 See ibid.

drawal of people from the study and the consequent change of therapies.

Ultimately, the efficacy of the vaccine for the purposes of Pfizer emergency authorization was not calculated based on death and other serious events (which were statistically insignificant), but on the 170 infected and on an alleged ability of the vaccine to decrease the possibility of contracting the infection by more than 30%. Yet the percentage of 170 infected out of the total number of study participants is less than zero. So it can be said that the vaccine was EUA approved based on statistics below zero and in reference to almost irrelevant numbers. This, I repeat, basically depends on the fact that the incidence of Covid-19 on the target population is not significant in terms of adverse effects and mortality, and has a minimal significance compared to the raw data of the infections.

5.1.3.2.1. Vaccine Efficacy and Communication Fraud

The anti-Covid vaccines under emergency authorization were presented to the public as having an extraordinary efficacy, exceeding 90%. The Pfizer vaccine, for example, was touted as 95% effective.[94] This was reassuring news to everyone. The effect was to lead people to think that, in the face of the terrible danger of the pandemic, these miraculous products could provide almost complete protection, leaving just a 5% risk.

In light of what was said in the previous section, we are now able to understand why this news involved true communi-

94 Cfr., ad es., EMA, "Comirnaty – Public Assessment Report," 23/12/2020, URL: https://www.ema.europa.eu/en/documents/assessment-report/comirnaty-epar-public-assessment-report_en.pdf; FDA, "Comirnaty and Pfizer-BioNTech COVID-19 Vaccine - Emergency Use Authorization (EUA) for an Unapproved Product, Decision Memorandum," December 11, 2020, URL: https://www.fda.gov/media/144416/download.

cation fraud against the whole world that was unaware of the pro-vaccine technicalities. The 95% efficacy rate, in fact, was not calculated with respect to the virus or disease, but with respect to the number of infections in the population subjected to the pre-authorization studies. Of that ridiculously low number of infected people (170 out of about 44,000), 8 belonged to the placebo group and 168 to that of the vaccinated. Thus, it was said numerically that compared to the two groups, the efficacy of the vaccine was 95%. However, this percentage—which, as we have already seen, did not address among other things serious adverse events and deaths—could in no way convey the real sense of the efficacy of these products in the fight against the pandemic and in personal protection.

Let's try to look at this from other points of view that are more suitable for real and honest evaluation. The pre-authorization studies (with data similar to those of other documents such as Report 9) showed that out of the unvaccinated population of 18,379, only 168 had become infected (about 0.9%) while out of the vaccinated population of 18,242, only 8 had become infected (about 0.04%). If we call not vaccinating "NV" and getting vaccinated "V," we could therefore say that "NV" protects from contagion at about 99.1% while "V" protects against contagion at 99.96%. "V" therefore, compared to the pandemic, improves the contagion situation compared to "NV" by 0.86%. Neither "NV" nor "V" can be said to protect against serious consequences or death from Covid-19. Regarding "V," however, we do not know any future or potential adverse effects, because the experimental testing on this product has just begun. Thus, for a marginal advantage of 0.86%, one would have to accept the unknown and unpredictable risk of the effects of the vaccine. This is a more understandable way of speaking for those who, from the outside, must be able to evaluate their pros and cons with respect to these new products.

Let me give you an analogical example in order to better understand where the communication scam lies. Imagine that a construction engineer tries to sell you a new type of brick or lime or mortar, saying that its use will protect your home from hurricanes 95% of the time. At this point, based on the tempting idea that, with this building novelty, your house will have only a 5% risk of being destroyed by a hurricane, you agree to spend the necessary money and give your ok to a renovation project. What would you have done, though, if you had been told that your home was already 99.1% hurricane-safe and that the new material would give you a marginal increase in protection of only 0.86% against an unpredictable risk of damage to the very structure of the house? To say that only a madman would agree to renovate a house under these conditions is an understatement. But here we are! This is what has happened with the pro-vaccine propaganda for emergency authorizations, and it is what is also happening these days with the current vaccine propaganda for imposing the vaccine on children.

5.1.3.3. "Unknown Benefits": Official Documents Have Always Said So

As I previously stated, there is no need to trust the words of Tal Zaks, Peter Doshi, Eric Topol, or any other scholar or expert on the subject in these matters. Just read what was written about these vaccines in the initial FDA documents.

On December 10, 2020, when the FDA Advisory Committee was to meet to evaluate the approval of the Pfizer vaccine (the first, as we know, to be approved), the FDA prepared a detailed study (a briefing document) to allow Committee members to study the facts of the matter.[95] Chapter eight of this study deals with the benefit-risk assessment and details all known and unknown benefits and risks of the vaccine.

The first section on known benefits is short and reassuring. It basically says that a high efficacy was found "in preventing

95 See ibid. All quotes in this paragraph are from this document and the underlines are mine.

PCR confirmed COVID-19 occurring at least 7 days after completion of the vaccination regimen." The efficacy of the first dose cannot be assessed because the second dose was administered within three weeks, not providing sufficient time to observe the consequences.

However, this section is followed by several other sections on unknown benefits and data gaps.

1. Duration of Protection

   "As the interim and final analyses have a limited length of follow-up, it is not possible to assess sustained efficacy over a period longer than 2 months."

   The duration of the studies is therefore too limited to be able to affirm protection of more than two months.

   For me, this is enough to question the entire emergency authorization for a logistical reason. Any mass vaccination of the population cannot be completed in two months, with the consequence that the effort employed can theoretically be nullified by the simultaneous loss of efficacy of the product. It's like trying to fill a sieve, so to speak.

2. Immunocompromised

   "The subset of certain groups such as immunocompromised individuals (e.g., those with HIV/AIDS) is too small to evaluate efficacy outcomes."

   Here the data are insufficient for an assessment. As relates to these subjects, any benefits of the vaccine are purely conjectural. Stakeholders should be warned of this, and doctors should tell them that they have no scientific basis for giving a well-founded opinion.

3. Individuals with prior infection

"Available data are insufficient to make conclusions about benefit in individuals with prior SARS-CoV-2 infection."

Here too the data are insufficient. In the case of these individuals, any benefits of the vaccine are purely conjectural. Stakeholders should be warned of this, and doctors should tell them that they have no scientific basis for giving a well-founded opinion.

4. Pediatric population

"The representation of pediatric participants in the study population is too limited to adequately evaluate efficacy in pediatric age groups younger than 16 years [...] it is biologically reasonable to extrapolate that effectiveness in ages 16 to 17 years would be similar to effectiveness in younger adults."

Here, too, there is insufficient data for evaluation.

It should also be noted that for individuals over 16 years of age, the efficacy of the vaccine is not based upon experimental science, but is the result of mere theoretical conjecture.

5. Evolution of the pandemic

"The study enrollment and follow-up occurred during the period of July 27 to November 14, 2020, in various geographical locations. The evolution of the pandemic characteristics, such as increased attack rates, increased exposure of subpopulations, as well as potential changes in the virus infectivity, antigenically significant mutations to the S protein, and/or the effect of coinfections may potentially limit the generalizability of the efficacy conclusions over time."

Therefore, anything could happen to change the parameters of efficacy and safety envisaged over time.

This, for me, as someone who always looks at things from a legal perspective, is a safeguard clause made precisely in light of the almost ridiculous duration of the provisional testing times used for the purposes of emergency authorization, times ranging from July to November: five months compared to the normal period of five years. The FDA is essentially telling us that, given the ridiculous observation time used, anything could happen, with respect to the trend of the epidemic, capable of changing the parameters of risks and benefits observed on the vaccine.

6. Asymptomatic infection

   "Data are limited to assess the effect of the vaccine against asymptomatic infection as measured by detection of the virus and/or detection of antibodies against non-vaccine antigens that would indicate infection rather than an immune response induced by the vaccine."

   Once again, evaluation is impossible due to lack of sufficient data.

   This figure, in this specific case, is astounding for anyone with a reasonable approach to the matter. The impossibility of assessing the efficacy of the vaccine on the asymptomatic population alone is an almost insurmountable obstacle to marketing authorization because it makes the results of the vaccine's use completely uncertain and unpredictable.

7. Long-term efficacy on the effects of Covid

"COVID-19 disease may have long-term effects on certain organs, and at present it is not possible to assess whether the vaccine will have an impact on specific long-term sequelae of COVID-19 disease in individuals who are infected despite vaccination. Demonstrated high efficacy against symptomatic COVID-19 should translate to overall prevention of COVID-19- related sequelae in vaccinated populations, though it is possible that asymptomatic infections may not be prevented as effectively as symptomatic infections and may be associated with sequelae that are either late-onset or undetected at the time of infection (e.g., myocarditis)."

Basically, if one becomes infected despite vaccination, the vaccine does not necessarily protect him from the effects of the disease. Now, if we consider this data together with those on the temporal limitation (two months) of the efficacy found based on the studies, and that on the statistical irrelevance of serious events among the participants, we understand how this contrasts with the entire media and political propaganda that the vaccine protects against severe consequences of the disease. The initial study clearly states that there was no data to support such a claim.

8. Efficacy on mortality

"A larger number of individuals at high risk of COVID-19 and higher attack rates would be needed to confirm efficacy of the vaccine against mortality. However, non-COVID vaccines (e.g., influenza) that are efficacious against disease have also been shown to prevent disease associated death. Benefits in preventing death should be evaluated in large observational studies following authorization."

There are therefore no data available to evaluate the vaccine's efficacy in preventing deaths. I must also point out two things about this FDA specification.

The first is the conjectural reference to traditional vaccines, which not only is not based upon experimental science and is of very little value in itself (given the generic level of conjecture involved), but is also scientifically fallacious given that anti-Covid vaccines use a new technology never utilized before, and with respect to which, therefore, conjectural similarities cannot be made with other different products. This error will appear more clearly in light of what I will say later on the notion of vaccines. Traditional vaccines are not vaccines in the same (illogical) way in which anti-Covid vaccines have been defined as such. If, with a logical leap, someone first gives the same name to different things and then, on the basis of this same name, elaborates a conjectural similarity between the two things, he makes a logical mistake of such magnitude that it does not even deserve to be heard.

The second thing concerns the postponement of subsequent studies, which logically expresses the fact that experimentation on this aspect is not yet sufficient and must be continued in the period following the marketing of the vaccine.

9. Efficacy on the transmission of the virus

"Data are limited to assess the effect of the vaccine against transmission of SARS-CoV-2 from individuals who are infected despite vaccination. Demonstrated high efficacy against symptomatic COVID-19 may translate to overall prevention of transmission in populations with high enough vaccine uptake, though it is possible that if effica-

> cy against asymptomatic infection were lower than efficacy against symptomatic infection, asymptomatic cases in combination with reduced mask-wearing and social distancing could result in significant continued transmission. Additional evaluations including data from clinical trials and from vaccine use post-authorization will be needed to assess the effect of the vaccine in preventing virus shedding and transmission, in particular in individuals with asymptomatic infection."
>
> Here too there are no data for an evaluation, and the scientific need to continue experimentation after authorization clearly emerges.
>
> The uncertainty relating to asymptomatic patients and, above all, the uncertainty regarding the protection of the vaccine should also be noted. The available data suggests that you can get infected despite the vaccine and that you can infect others. Once again, the difference between technical data and political media propaganda is stark.
>
> Furthermore, the uncertainty about asymptomatic people means that this vaccine cannot be used to promote policies to mitigate other prevention measures (masks, distancing, etc.) which has instead been done by many authorities in many countries.

The EMA, which obviously uses the same FDA data for Pfizer, concludes its analysis on the clinical efficacy of the vaccine for the purposes of conditional marketing authorization by saying that an "excellent vaccine efficacy" of 95% was found (which I already refuted above) in preventing "symptomatic COVID-19," and thus summarizes the other aspects of efficacy that I have just reported from the section on "unknown benefits" (which I have stylistically taken from the FDA but which naturally coincides with what is reported by the EMA):

> "It is likely that the vaccine also protects against severe COVID-19, though these events were rare in the study, and statistically certain conclusions cannot be drawn. It is presently not known if the vaccine protects against asymptomatic infection, or its impact on viral transmission. The duration of protection is not known.
>
> The CHMP [Committee for Medicinal Products for Human Use] considers the following measures necessary to address the missing efficacy data in the context of a conditional MA [Marketing Authorization]: The final clinical study report will be submitted no later than December 2023 and is subject to a specific obligation laid down in the MA. This will provide long-term data."[96]

In this conclusion, the references to excellent efficacy and the likelihood that the vaccine will protect against the serious consequences of the disease are misleading. The postponement to the testing phase in progress for missing data confirms the ongoing testing inherent in the emergency authorization.[97] And the other unknown aspects (which are also reported in the indications of the EMA for the general public) reveal the discrepancy between the real technical data and the manipulation of that data by the mainstream media and politics. On the basis of these data (which have never changed),[98] for example, neither the green pass poli-

---

96 See, e.g., EMA, "Comirnaty – Public Assessment Report," op. cit., p. 97.

97 This technical reference to the studies in progress, of course, is repeated at various points in the relevant documents. See, e.g., ibid, p. 94: "Overall, the study report including the final analysis is considered adequate. This is not the final report for the study, as the study is expected to continue for a total of 24 months."

98 See, e.g., EMA, "Comirnaty," Overview, January 21, 2022, URL: https://www.ema.europa.eu/en/medicines/human/EPAR/comirnaty#

(continued on the next page)

cies nor any hypothesis of mandatory vaccination can be justified.

Ultimately, we must ask ourselves, not only in general whether it was legitimate or appropriate to define as vaccines drugs that do not confer immunity from the disease, but also whether the emergency authorizations were really justified by any appreciable efficacy of the products in question. We must then ask ourselves whether, in an adequate and credible ethical and scientific system, the authorizations of these products should be suspended or withdrawn in light of the current scarce and increasingly unpredictable effectiveness that has been found. From an ethical point of view, we must ask ourselves whether the public has been illegitimately deceived into believing that these products had abundant experimental results (never before seen in the history of pharmacology!) thanks to the participation in clinical trials of tens of thousands of people. From my point of view, this was one of the biggest communication frauds in history, as well as an unprecedented global violation of the right to informed consent.

5.1.3.4. Vaccine Efficacy and Adverse Effects

Another very serious problem is also linked to efficacy from both an epidemiological and an ethical point of view: that is, the actual ability of the current system to distinguish between the positive and negative effects of vaccines. Agencies around the world are constantly giving updates comparing hospitalizations, intensive care and deaths of unvaccinated and vaccinated people

---

authorisation-details-section: "The impact of vaccination with Comirnaty on the spread of the SARS-CoV-2 virus in the community is not yet known. It is not yet known how much vaccinated people may still be able to carry and spread the virus [...] It is not currently known how long protection given by Comirnaty lasts. The people vaccinated in the clinical trial will continue to be followed for 2 years to gather more information on the duration of protection."

(with one, two or three doses). But are these data scientifically reliable?

First of all, it must be said that an effect of arbitrariness and fanaticism that has been generated on the subject has caused individual hospitals to adopt different and scientifically unfounded criteria from time to time to classify hospitalized patients as respectively vaccinated or unvaccinated. Recently, for example, an Italian academic and hospital director, stated that in his hospital (unlike others) people with double doses taken more than four months previously were classified as unvaccinated. It goes without saying that countless news items like this have occurred around the world, generating a generic unreliability of the aggregate data of the various government agencies. If hospitals send data that are unreliable or based on changing criteria, the agencies' statistical conclusions will be equally unreliable.

The most important thing that I would like to emphasize, however, does not concern the unpredictable arbitrariness of individuals, but the official criteria used by many agencies. In fact, it has been common to consider unvaccinated those who had received the dose of the vaccine within 14 or 15 days from the onset of Covid (that is, with a positive diagnosis of the disease). This criterion was adopted on the assumption that the efficacy of the vaccine does not operate immediately after administration but after a certain number of days later. This, for example, is the official criterion used by the Italian Institute of Health (ISS):

> "**Unvaccinated cases:** All cases reported with a confirmed diagnosis of SARS-CoV-2 virus infection that:
>
> - have not received any vaccine dose, or
> - have been vaccinated with either first dose or single dose vaccine within 14 days prior to diagnosis, or who have contracted the infection before the time necessary to

develop at least a partial immune response to the vaccine."[99]

Now, the first criterion is indubitable due to its evident relationship with observable reality. The second indicates, however, that the data of the unvaccinated also include adverse effects from the vaccine, which generally seem to be more serious if close to inoculation. In other words, if a person receives the vaccine dose and, within the next 14 days goes to intensive care or dies, he is considered an unvaccinated inpatient or Covid death. However, the question remains whether he was hospitalized or died from Covid or from the vaccine.

The truth is that until there are sufficient disaggregated data to distinguish between adverse effects of the vaccine, on the one hand, and the effects of Covid on the unvaccinated, on the other, it will not be possible to assess the impact of Covid on health conditions, hospitalizations, and deaths of the unvaccinated.

However, this would imply an active pharmacovigilance that politicians, violating a serious moral—but also legal—duty which, as I said, is stronger in the case of emergency drug authorizations, did not want to undertake. The reasons why politicians have chosen to violate this duty are not clear and, therefore, the lack of adequate active pharmacovigilance is even more suspicious.

Consequently, the only certain criterion at the moment, in the absence of adequate active pharmacovigilance and adequate disaggregated data, remains the first: that is, to simply distinguish between those who have never received any dose of the vaccine and those who have received it. However, such a criterion would

99 See ISS, "Epidemia COVID-19 - Aggiornamento nazionale 5 gennaio 2022," January 07, 2022, URL: https://www.epicentro.iss.it/coronavirus/bollettino/Bollettino-sorveglianza-integrata-COVID-19_5-gennaio-2022.pdf.

not be in favor of the vaccine and has generally been rejected. The moral (and theological) imperative seems to have been the "*favor vaccini*" at all costs until now. However, this is neither a correct scientific criterion nor an acceptable ethical criterion and should be strongly questioned by the scientific community and disregarded by politicians.

5.2. Diachronic Evaluation

Let me remind the reader that each of the assumptions of the emergency authorizations must be evaluated both in a synchronic and diachronic sense. The initial ethical choice of emergency authorization is justified if, in fact, at the time when those assumptions are made, they reasonably exist. Each of them, however, by its very nature, changes over time, sometimes in a sudden and intense way.

There are not a few, for example, who believe that today, at least in some countries, the conditions for a state of emergency are no longer present and that the numbers and risks of Covid have now dropped to the level of seasonal flu. Some countries have *de facto* or *de jure* canceled the state of emergency. With regard to the adverse effects, think for example of the suspension of the Moderna vaccine in Finland under the age of 30 and in Norway and Sweden under the age of 18,[100] or even the AstraZeneca case to which I will return in detail later.

5.3. Opposing and Conflicting Interests

Concerning all these presuppositions, it is also necessary to better understand the dynamics of the interests at stake. Pharma-

100 See M. Paterlini, "Covid-19: Sweden, Norway, and Finland suspend use of Moderna vaccine in young people 'as a precaution'," *BMJ* 2021, 375, n2477, doi:10.1136/bmj.n2477.

ceutical companies, in fact, have an inherent interest in ensuring that these elements remain in existence. Their best business depends on authorizations, and, from this point of view, it is good for them (so to speak) that the state of emergency persists, that vaccines are constantly linked to a certain efficacy in the fight against the epidemic, that there are no health system alternative means of reaction, that the fear of a serious fatal disease remains in the community, that the negative effects always appear lower than the positive ones, etc.

The political community and citizens, on the other hand, should be interested in the exact opposite. I use the conditional with respect to the political community because if we also include the government authorities, then the situation becomes more complicated or gray. Politics in power, in fact, draws several advantages from the state of emergency, which fact generates a conflict of interest that is intertwined in various ways with that of the pharmaceutical companies. Given the ability of pharmaceutical companies and politics to control public information, these conflicts of interest generate enormous doubts of an ethical nature that require extreme caution especially when evaluating sources and reliability of the news.[101]

These conflicts of interest, of course, would require a very strong balance of economic and political power on the part of journalism, especially with regard to information on vaccines and the preconditions for political decisions. The mainstream media, however, have aligned themselves with political propaganda favorable to the pharmaceutical industry in a very serious ethical violation of their proper role in the institutional democratic order. In Italy, during the pandemic, the state's public funding for newspapers doubled, which reveals a huge conflict of

101 This is the underlying theme of my work, *The Death of the Phronimos: Faith and Truth About anti-Covid Vaccines*, op. cit.

interest and explains why the media held a pro-government attitude towards vaccine policies.[102]

5.4. The Strange Science of Anti-Covid Vaccines

For my purposes, at this moment, I want to focus on just two of the aspects of emergency authorizations that I have summarized above. One is that the authorizations were granted based on provisional or incomplete data and therefore imply a developing experimental science that must continue to study and *experiment* after the authorizations are granted. In fact, both the FDA and the EMA, in compliance with the emergency regulations, require manufacturers to continue their trials and data collection in the post-authorization phase. The other is that the authorizations are granted based on the data and studies provided by the pharmaceutical companies themselves. Even for post-authorization studies, manufacturers always remain primarily responsible, despite being in conflict of interest with respect to the "science" of vaccines.

Some, thinking about the existence of government agencies on drugs such as the FDA and EMA, may imagine a *scientific* process directed and promoted by these public bodies, which perhaps take the initiative of sector studies or focus mainly, and with a scientific method, on the specific literature existing in the world of research. This is not quite the case. The real world of independent research cannot do anything in the pre-authorization phase and can do very little even afterwards, both

102 See, e.g., S. Cannavò, "Il finanziamento pubblico ai giornali è raddoppiato," *Il Fatto Quotidiano*, December 29, 2021, URL: https://www.ilfattoquotidiano.it/in-edicola/articoli/2021/12/29/il-finanziamento-pubblico-ai-giornali-e-raddoppiato/6439851/. On the relationship between politics and mainstream journalism with respect to anti Covid vaccines, I refer again to my work, *The Death of the Phronimos: Faith and Truth About anti-Covid Vaccines*, op. cit.

because it has less research funding and capacity than pharmaceutical companies and because it does not have all the relevant data and information, since many vaccines are protected as trade secrets.[103]

The very innovative mRNA and viral vector techniques are private assets or know-how of the companies that are developing them, and not freely available to public research bodies or universities. From this point of view, the reference to "science" in the field of Covid vaccines is highly ambiguous. Here "science" is above all the private one of pharmaceutical companies and is in a constant conflict of interests with the common good and with that of patients. The FDA, the CDC, or the EMA, after authorization, certainly have a great coordination capacity in the national collection of data on the use of vaccines and give important indications on the type of clinical studies and analyzes that are still needed, but they do not do the basic research of these studies and tests or trials themselves, which always leads to an imbalance between pharmaceutical companies and independent science.[104]

Let's go back to the pre-authorization phase. When a pharmaceutical company applies for emergency or conditional authorization for the use of a drug or vaccine, there is no scientific literature relating to it precisely because it is a new product. The pharmaceutical company, therefore, will apply to the responsible body with an application accompanied by its studies and clinical tests, and these documents (prepared by subjects in conflict of interest and scientifically not independent) will be the

103 On the recent FOIA appeal for administrative access to the FDA documents relating to the authorization of the Pfizer vaccine, see my book, *The Death of the Phronimos: Faith and Truth About anti-Covid Vaccines*, op. cit.

104 On these aspects too, and on the way of understanding the reference to "science" in the path leading to the approval of new drugs I speak specifically and extensively in *The Death of the Phronimos: Faith and Truth About anti-Covid Vaccines*, op. cit.

only ones that the relevant bodies will initially have available to evaluate whether to grant permission. If the application is credible, authorization will be granted. If not, the application will be rejected. In both cases, there is no scientific community involvement in this phase, except in the indirect sense that the assessments on the applications are made by experts from interested or relevant sectors.

Even after the emergency authorizations have been granted, the independent studies of the scientific community will largely depend on the data on vaccines and tests that the pharmaceutical companies (or the entities in charge) will gradually make available. It is obvious, however, that after the marketing of a product, many other data will be collected, generated in a way that is wholly or partly independent of the pharmaceutical companies, and through which science in a broad sense can express itself. The basic concept, in any case, is that emergency approved vaccines are not a sector in which the reference to "science" has a unique and acceptable meaning for common sense and public opinion.

The comparison between the explanations of the authorizations offered by the two main agencies constantly referenced by the world mass media (the FDA and the EMA) also makes it clear that we must look at substantive and not at nominalistic issues. These two agencies do similar work, and the common goal, in times of emergency, is to make available a drug or vaccine that otherwise would not have yet been in scientific and safe conditions to be used. The FDA authorizes the use of "unapproved" vaccines in an emergency. The EMA conditionally "approves" vaccines that have no medical alternatives. Those who discuss whether or not vaccines are "approved" on the basis of these nominalistic legal differences have not understood the substance of the matter and will always remain ambiguous with respect to the international scenario. The main common criteria are the ones I have listed above: the state of emergency, a life-threatening disease, the lack of alternatives, the prevalence of positive expectations over unknown risks, etc. The common goal is that these criteria be respected in the best possible way.

5.5. Informed Consent

The FDA has an extremely clear formula on the consequences of emergency authorization with regard to disclosure and consent:

> "How will vaccine recipients be informed about the benefits and risks of any vaccine that receives an EUA [Emergency Use Authorization]?
> FDA must ensure that recipients of the vaccine under an EUA are informed, to the extent practicable given the applicable circumstances, that FDA has authorized the emergency use of the vaccine, of the known and potential benefits and risks, the extent to which such benefits and risks are unknown, that they have the option to accept or refuse the vaccine, and of any available alternatives to the product. Typically, this information is communicated in a patient "fact sheet." The FDA posts these fact sheets on our website."[105]

The European law on conditional authorizations contains a similar indication dependent on the assumption that it is

105 See U.S. Food and Drug Administration, "Emergency Use Authorization for Vaccines Explained," URL:, https://www.fda.gov/vaccines-blood-biologics/vaccines/emergency-use-authorization-vaccines-explained. The underlines are mine. In one of the first meetings of the FDA Advisory Committee, that of December 10, 2020, it was already stressed that the nature of the authorization required to clarify, through the fact sheets, both to those who administer the vaccine and to those who receive the vaccine, the "investigational nature of the product," see https://www.fda.gov/emergency-preparedness-and-response/coronavirus-disease-2019-covid-19/covid-19-vaccines#meetings.

an authorization that has altered the normal scientific procedure on the testing and evaluation of drugs.

> "Clear information should be provided to patients and healthcare professionals on the conditional nature of the authorisations. It is therefore necessary that such information be clearly stated in the summary of product characteristics of the medicinal product concerned as well as on the package leaflet."[106]
>
> "Where a medicinal product has been granted conditional marketing authorisation in accordance with this Regulation, the information included in the summary of product characteristics and package leaflet shall contain a clear mention of that fact. The summary of product characteristics shall also contain the date on which the conditional authorisation is due for renewal."[107]

Here it is important to note the technical way in which this type of emergency authorization requires both the need for clear information on the nature of the authorization and for freedom of choice to be ensured to those who potentially receive the drug. How could it be otherwise? Knowing about the emergency vaccine regime takes priority over all other specific information. This proves that this is a circumstance which, although intertwined with the other assumptions and traits of the emergency authorization, possesses its own crucial autonomy for the purposes of ethical reasoning. For the moral agent, it is important to know about the state of emergency even earlier and regardless of knowing its more specific characteristics.

We need to be extremely clear on this point. If there was no emergency authorization, the use of the drug or vaccine in question would continue according to the legislation on the testing of pharmaceutical products on humans and would require patients to voluntarily undergo experimental medical treatment.

---

106 See Reg. (CE) n. 507/2006, op. cit., point "(10)."

107 Ibid. art. 8.

If an average of five years is foreseen for the experimentation of a drug, this means that during these five years all those who use the drug in question participate as “volunteers” in scientific medical research. If for an emergency reason the law decides to cut or shorten the ordinary course of scientific experimentation, it must at the same time ensure that whoever uses the drug in question is made aware of the substance of the situation: that is, of the fact that the drug is in emergency use, or that, in the absence of the exceptional legal measure, its regular experimentation would still be in progress.

The voluntary nature of participating in a trial on human beings must therefore be replaced by the informed consent of the emergency legislation. If this information is not provided adequately, a person is being subjected to experimental treatment in a deceptive way and without his consent. I will return to this point again later.

5.5.1. From Technical “may be” to Deceptive Certainty

Peter Doshi pointed out to me a technical terminological issue of emergency authorization documents which, for my ethical purposes, is of crucial importance. It’s about the use of the term “may be.”

The documents of the emergency authorizations, precisely because they are based on the interruption of the ordinary and normal path of experimental drug science, imply a technical judgment on the efficacy of a hypothetical nature. Certainty cannot be provided when the path of science is still in progress, *in itinere*, in execution. The judgments on safety, on the other hand, albeit provisional, need greater certainty. You can't tell people to take a drug that “may be” safe. As I explained earlier, the risk-benefit ratio, as a requirement for emergency authorizations, must be positive. As for efficacy, however, all the FDA emergency authorization documents for the anti-Covid vaccines carry the technical expression "may be." Let's read them all:

> "Based on the totality of scientific evidence available, including data from adequate and well-controlled trials described in Section 4 of this review, it is reasonable to believe that the Pfizer-BioNTech COVID-19 vaccine (BNT162b2) may be effective in preventing such serious or life-threatening disease or condition that can be caused by SARS-CoV-2."[108]
>
> "Based on the totality of scientific evidence available, including data from adequate and well-controlled trials described in Section 4 of this review, it is reasonable to believe that the Moderna COVID-19 vaccine (mRNA-1273) may be effective in preventing such serious or life-threatening disease or condition that can be caused by SARS-CoV-2."[109]
>
> "Based on the totality of scientific evidence available, including data from adequate and well-controlled trials described in Section 4 of this review, it is reasonable to

108 See FDA, Comirnaty and Pfizer-BioNTech COVID-19 Vaccine, "Decision Memorandum," op. cit., p. 55.

109 See FDA, Moderna COVID-19 Vaccine, "Decision Memorandum," December 18, 2020, URL: https://www.fda.gov/media/144673/download, p. 60. See, also, FDA News Release, "FDA Takes Additional Action in Fight Against COVID-19 By Issuing Emergency Use Authorization for Second COVID-19 Vaccine," December 18, 2020, URL: https://www.fda.gov/news-events/press-announcements/fda-takes-additional-action-fight-against-covid-19-issuing-emergency-use-authorization-second-covid: "The totality of the available data provides clear evidence that the Moderna COVID-19 Vaccine may be effective in preventing COVID-19. The data also show that the known and potential benefits outweigh the known and potential risks." Note here the difference in terminology between the judgments of efficacy and safety, but also the fact that the safety judgment is also expressed with respect to potential risks, which, as we know, implies an impossible and conjectural evaluation.

believe that the Janssen COVID-19 vaccine may be effective in preventing such a serious or life-threatening disease or condition that can be caused by SARS-CoV-2."[110]

All the technical documents say (correctly) that the drug could be effective, using terminology that conceptually recalls the very meaning of emergency authorizations in the face of experimental science in progress. This terminology is also properly in line with the qualified informed consent required by the nature of emergency authorizations (which we have just revisited). The use of the "may be" already reveals *per se* the existence of scientific uncertainty relating to the drug and indicates the need for special consent from those who may face the option of taking it. Not using "may be," by any public authority or journalist, is already a serious violation of informed consent.

Needless to say, information on these vaccines occurred at all levels in the name of an alleged scientific certainty about their efficacy; so evident (it has been said in all sorts of ways) to overcome any doubt and accusation from "ignorant critics, fanatics, terrorists, sewer rats," etc. etc., that is, all those who continued to have doubts and/or to voice them. Even government agencies and drug agencies around the world have almost always listed these pseudo-vaccines as *safe and effective* in public information without further qualification. This gives the idea of the disproportionate extent of immorality that has unfortunately characterized the entire public debate on these experimental products since they were put on the market.

110 See FDA, Janssen COVID-19 Vaccine, "Decision Memorandum," February 27, 2021, p. 64, URL: https://www.fda.gov/media/146338/download.

Chapter 6

The Epistemology and Ethics of Emergency Authorizations

In this chapter, I will not analyze the specific legal and ethical assumptions of emergency authorizations. This is something that I will have to do elsewhere since these assumptions constitute, each of them, as many circumstances of vaccines as are relevant both to public ethics and to individual ethics. Here I propose to address the overall epistemological and ethical sense of the very existence of emergency authorizations.

This chapter, therefore, like the previous ones, has an architectural ethical role. Moral conscience, even before going into the ethical and normative details of emergency authorizations, must become aware of the overall panorama in which they take on meaning and be able to evaluate it as such. From this point of view, it is important both to offer general clarifications on the meaning of the authorizations in question and to reflect on the actual context in which they operate. I must therefore focus specifically on the essential aspects of an epistemological, ethical, and legal nature. Subsequently, I will continue the discussion by retracing the narrative context of the most salient facts that characterized above all the AstraZeneca case, the definitive approval of the Pfizer vaccine, and some subsequent events politically and scientifically linked to it. Sometimes, nothing helps the moral conscience more than focusing on how some concrete facts and debates have unfolded.

6.1. The Epistemological Profile of Emergency Authorizations

The information just mentioned at the end of the previous chapter reveals the link between the underlying epistemological aspect of emergency authorizations and their ethical consequences. As far as the science of current Covid vaccines is concerned, the authorizations mean a very important thing: that this science is not certain, safe, stable, and/or properly tested. Citizens must be informed of this. Emergency authorization means accelerated and less thorough processes; it means provisional science. Emergency authorization is the law that determines the rules and limits of the use of a drug that is still in the trial phase.

What happens with these authorizations is that the law, being aware of the intrinsic characteristics and meaning of its own emergency processes (which force or compress science in the face of necessity), requires people to be aware of the reduced truth value of science concerning anti-Covid vaccines; a reduced value which is intrinsic to these vaccines. As I have already said, the legal sense of emergency authorizations (whatever they are called in the specific regulatory systems) is to incorporate within itself—that is, within the legal procedure or the sphere of law—the remaining phase of experimentation and scientific evaluation of a product. This product, used urgently by decision of the political authority before being scientifically ready, will still have to continue its scientific path, but it will do so under the aegis and control of the same law that anticipated its use. This is something that the law knows and that, consequently, citizens must know. Law knows the difference between itself and science, and ensures that science remains that—science—even when it has to take place or develop within a context of political decisions and legal controls.

The epistemology of emergency authorizations concerns firstly, their nature and overall legal meaning that we have just revisited and, secondly, the interpretation and truth evaluation of the specific assumptions that legitimize them.

6.2. The Ethical Importance of Emergency Authorizations

Returning to our general discourse on the circumstances of the moral act, it is clear that this type of authorizations (with all that they objectively entail) is extremely important for the ethical subject who approaches the choice of vaccinating or not vaccinating. It is also quite evident that the context of these authorizations entails a state of serious doubt about the consequences of vaccines for one's health. Indeed, it involves considerable unknowns and *gambles*, and therefore requires enormous respect for everyone's freedom.

The fact that many governments, experts, and journalists have tried to belittle, and almost hide, the objective meaning of these authorizations is already highly immoral *per se*. Regarding them and vaccines in general, if anything, the attitude of everyone, and especially of those who have privileged access to the media, should be focused on creating an environment of maximum transparency and respect. Doubts must first *be generated* based on correct information so that it is clear to everyone that they exist. This is what information is for! Then they must be taken seriously and respected in the concrete choices of any individual. Those who do not do so show a very mediocre ethical and political sensitivity.

The reason why I addressed this circumstance separately from the previous one (on the uncertainties of medium and long-term negative effects) is that, in the conscience of the moral subject, it clearly has an importance *per se*. The mere fact of knowing the legal meaning of these emergency authorizations (let's call them all that, including those of the EMA, for simplicity and substantive truth) puts the moral agent on the alert even before and independently from reflecting on other specific issues concerning vaccines and the epidemic.

Naturally, the issues on anti-Covid vaccines are all intertwined, but the circumstance of authorizations has its own autonomy because it mainly concerns a legal aspect, while the circumstance on short, medium, or long-term doubts mainly concerns a medical-scientific aspect. The FDA and the EMA are government agencies. Technically, their decision has a legal nature (even if it is mostly based on medical data). When one of these agencies makes a decision within the sphere of its competence, the citizen can legitimately assume that the authority in charge has deemed it had sufficient elements for that decision. Epistemologically it remains a juridical decision, albeit based above all (but not only) on medical scientific evaluations.

The circumstance of the effects and risks, as such, is instead substantial and is based solely on one's understanding of the unknowns about vaccines. For the purposes of this understanding, government agencies are just one of the sources to turn to. In other words, knowing about the emergency authorization immediately tells the citizen that there are strong doubts but that, given the state of emergency, the authority is acting exceptionally by deviating from the normal rules of medical, scientific, and political prudence. Reflecting on the effects and risks of vaccines for the purposes of one's own moral assessments, on the other hand, goes beyond the mere knowledge of legal and political decisions. It goes in the direction of a substantial knowledge of the issues at stake to be satisfied with any available tool.

6.2.1. But the Vaccine Has Been Given to Billions of People

I now want to touch upon the objection that the current Covid vaccines are not experimental anymore because they have by now been administered to billions of people. This objection has had some media success and *prima facie* has a certain conceptual appeal to the general public. How can one say that a drug that has had such an extensive field trial is still experimental? This type of objection is fallacious for many reasons, but it also has a crucial ethical consequence on which it is worth reflecting.

First of all, it is an objection that is based on a misunderstanding between the synchronic and diachronic aspects of experimentation. It is obvious, in fact, that, in the various experimental sciences, experiments capable of validating or verifying a theory or hypothesis must be adequate for the theory or hypothesis in question. From this point of view, it is natural that, with respect to potential harmful consequences of some products, the experiment must have synchronic intensity and diachronic duration proportionate to the standards that each individual science develops in order to give a reasonable degree of reliability to the results of the experiments themselves.

In pharmacological science, for example, the testing standards for new products are five years because this is the reasonable time within which positive or negative effects can be assessed. In other sciences, the timing can vary greatly also depending on the possibility of forcing the parameters of the experiment. The solidity and durability of a new building science material, for example, could be tested in the short term by subjecting it to anomalous tensions and temperatures; something that obviously cannot be done with human beings (at least not after the experiments of the Nazi doctors and the trial that condemned them). From this point of view, if a negative effect of a drug is destined to occur four years after administration, the fact of immediately administering the drug to a billion people only means that the negative effect in four years will be multiplied as a percentage by a billion people.

In my book *The Death of the Phronimos,*[111] I go over some recent scandals of pharmaceutical companies also to highlight the time needed for these scandals to come to light. The case

111 See F. Di Blasi, *The Death of the Phronimos: Faith and Truth about Anti Covid Vaccines*, op. cit.

of Vioxx seemed particularly illuminating to me because it took five years after authorization, an experimental study on more than 40,000 people, more than 60,000 deaths, and billions in compensation for the pharmaceutical company that produced it (and not the FDA!) to decide to withdraw it from the market. For the other details of this scandal and for a comparison with the current case of the extension of the Covid vaccine to children, I refer to that book.

In construction science, insufficiently tested materials have often been used, such as certain resins for grouting or non-alkali-resistant fiberglass nets to strengthen balconies. This second material, for example, has been found to lose its mechanical characteristics over the years by reacting with cement, pH, etc., with the consequence that balconies risk collapsing much earlier than expected. Just think, to take another analogical example, that in the case of roof terraces, the tested times of materials and techniques lead to a guarantee of good resistance of at least ten years. This means that if a terrace causes infiltrations or yields before ten years without the influence of events of an exceptional nature (such as earthquakes and hurricanes), a good lawyer will be able to obtain compensation for damages from the construction company or the construction manager. The law, in these cases, encodes the certainties of experimental science by generating legal and jurisprudential parameters of responsibility.

Now, hypothesize, as a thought experiment, that due to an emergency of some kind, the government of a country decides to approve the use of a new material not yet tested to build houses. Maybe there are many immigrants to host or extraterrestrials to be given political asylum. I'm kidding of course, but I'm doing it to better visualize this kind of thought experiment. Given the nature of the emergency and the government authorization, the construction industry works a real miracle and manages to build more than a billion new homes in less than a year using the experimental material approved in an emergency. At this point, faced with the doubts of the material's resistance expressed by some technicians, the experts of the government, of licensing agencies or of television cabarets react by saying that by now, after such a large-scale use of the material, it must be considered well tested. It is obvious that such a reaction is complete nonsense. If the new material was destined to create structural problems after, for example, three years, the only consequence of having used it for a billion homes is that, instead of a few collapsing, many will collapse. In the case of a drug like Vioxx, instead of a few people dying, more than 60,000 died.

6.2.2. The Number of Doses Administered Is Not Experimental Science

In addition to the diachronic fallacy of these objections, there is also one concerning the very nature of experimental science. In fact, giving someone the Covid vaccine does not in itself mean experimenting with it. As I have already pointed out, in the case of these vaccines, what is closest to experimental science is what happened in the pre-authorization phase with many volunteers and by pharmaceutical companies.

In this phase, despite having reduced the experimentation times from five years to less than one year, some tens of thousands of people were involved, and the double-blind system was adopted.[112] Therefore, even with the limitations and defects I already mentioned (shortening of the times, conflict of interest, secret data, impossibility of verification by medical science), we are in a theoretically suitable context for providing experimental results because we are hypothetically matching the parameters of experimental science applied to medicine. The problem remains of how reliable is an experimental datum that cannot be tested by independent science, but only reported by those who are in con-

112 We know by now that it was not a true double blind, but I will not dwell on this aspect here.

flict of interest with respect to the story itself.[113] In the abstract, however—for those who want to make this act of faith—it is possible to speak of experimental science. I repeat, it is an experimental science that has the diachronic limits which I have just mentioned, and the proof of this is the constant failure of any forecast of efficacy as well as the many negative effects added to the leaflets from month to month after the various products have been placed on the market. These effects have already resulted in the death and personal injury of many people. They are therefore not purely theoretical questions.

This is therefore the experimental science—limited and without certainty—of the pre-authorization period. Then there is the experimental science of the post-authorization period. I have already talked about this too, including, a) the underlying theoretical aspect that prevents us from considering purely statistical data as experimental data, b) the enormous limits of passive pharmacovigilance, and c) public and governmental ostracism towards reporting and study of adverse effects. Beyond these limits and defects, it must be clearly stated that in the proper sense, even in the post-authorization phase, experimental science is only that which occurs within the parameters of tests and clinical studies.

In fact, for the extension of the use of Covid vaccines to new population groups, such as children between 12 and 17 years and children between 5 and 11 years, experimental studies were conducted on a thousand children in the first case and just over two thousand in the second (not counting those who received the placebo). In general, almost all post-authorization experimental studies, also aimed at evaluating the efficacy of vaccines, have

113 See the recent appeal for transparency on Covid vaccine data that appeared on the pages of the *British Medical Journal*: P. Doshi, F. Godlee, K. Abbasi, "Covid-19 vaccines and treatments: we must have raw data now," *BMJ*, Published 19 January 2022, 376:o102, doi:10.1136/bmj.o102.

been carried out from time to time on a few hundred people. To those who do experimental science, of course, it is not enough to say that vaccines are used by billions of people to talk about experimental results. Each experimental result is such only and exclusively if conducted in the laboratory, so to speak, respecting all the parameters and monitoring systems required by the experimental science of the specific discipline. The reference to the billions of people is not done by experts among themselves, but by demagogues with populations to manipulate.

6.2.3. The Breaking of the Double Blind

Compared to the path of the experimental science of anti-Covid vaccines in the post-authorization phase, a huge problem that arose was the breaking of the double blind after the emergency authorization. This rupture deprived most of the tests launched in the pre-authorization phase of scientific sense. A serious and detached scientific discussion should be initiated on this because, if it is true that after authorization it would have been ethically difficult to prevent those who received the placebo from choosing to receive the vaccine, it is also true that giving this possibility of choice has damaged the experimental path of vaccines in a substantial and irreparable way.[114]

114 See, e.g., P.R. Krause, M.F. Gruber, "Emergency Use Authorization of Covid Vaccines - Safety and Efficacy Follow-Up Considerations," *The New England Journal of Medicine*, 2020 Nov 5, 383(19):e107, Published online on October 16, 2020, doi: 10.1056/NEJMp2031373: "The quality of the data available to inform ongoing assessment of a vaccine's benefits and risks will depend on the ability to continue evaluating the vaccine against a placebo comparator in clinical trials for as long as feasible. Moreover, evaluation of other potentially superior vaccines will depend on the ability to continue to maintain placebo controls in ongoing trials. Thus, issuance of an EUA should not, in and of itself, require unblinding of a Covid-19 vaccine trial and immediate vaccination of placebo recipients, since doing so may jeopardize approval of these products." See also

(continued on the next page)

From this point of view, the doubt must be raised that the emergency authorization was too premature, and therefore ethically wrong even for this precise issue. Is it possible that the emergency authorizations sacrificed experimental medical science in this case on the altar of the frenzy of politics in difficulty? And, of course, I am not thinking only of the difficulties related to the confrontation with the pandemic, but also of the difficulties of consensus and political stability of parties that needed to distract the attention of the population from their faults (such as, in the United States, with respect to Afghanistan and the illegal immigration crisis). The conflict of interest of the parties in power compared to the fear of the virus and the state of emergency is no less than the conflict of interest of the pharmaceutical companies compared to the billionaire business of the authorization of anti-Covid vaccines. Anyone who underestimates these aspects demonstrates a very poor epistemological capacity for legal ethical questions.

To be clear, I am not opposed to breaking the double blind in the interest of the patient when, of course, this is done on the basis of serious and well-argued considerations. It is natural that the interest in the patient's life and health cannot be annihilated by some sort of common good of the experiment. The breaking of the double blind, from this point of view, responds to a criterion opposite to the ethical utilitarianism that exploits

---

A. Rid, M. Lipsitch, F. G. Miller, "The Ethics of Continuing Placebo in SARS-CoV-2 Vaccine Trials," *JAMA*, 2021;325(3):219-220, Published Online on December 14, 2020, doi:10.1001/jama.2020.25053; P. Doshi, D. Light, "How to Expand Access to COVID Vaccines without Compromising the Science. Emergency Use Authorizations by the FDA Are Not Ideal," op. cit.; R. Dal-Ré, "US FDA Erratic Approach to Placebo-Controlled Trials after Issuing an Emergency Use Authorization for a COVID-19 Vaccine," Elsevier, Volume 39, Issue 8, February 22, 2021, Pages 1180-1182, Published online on January 20, 2021, doi: 10.1016/j.vaccine.2021.01.050.

the individual for the community. This is a similar criterion, for example, to that which makes it immoral to administer a potentially dangerous drug to a child in the interest of an elderly person.

However, it is necessary to reflect on the possible circularity or illogicality of the reasoning that leads to the breaking of the double blind in the case of emergency authorizations for anti-Covid vaccines. The safety and reliability of the emergency authorization is based on provisional data deriving from pre-authorization tests and studies. These data must be *verified* with the continuation of those tests and studies. The ethical requirement of breaking the double blind after authorization derives, on the other hand, from the idea that an authorized drug enjoys a medical advantage *verified* by the authorization itself and therefore must also be made available to those who had received the placebo. Here, however, the circularity appears. The additional scientific certainty of the emergency authorization depends, in fact, on those same studies whose results can be compromised by breaking the double blind. The ongoing experimental studies (which include the subjects who received the placebo) give a truth basis to the emergency authorization, and the emergency authorization gives a truth basis to the administration of the vaccine to those who are part of those studies. The studies *verify* the authorization that *verifies* the interruption of those studies.

Let's imagine testing a new type of resin to reinforce the buildings' floor structures and doing a double-blind experiment on a series of buildings using resin for only half of them and using traditional materials for the other half. The experiment is intended to last two years, but exceptionally it is decided that the partial results are such as to authorize the emergency use of the resin after only one year. On the basis of this authorization, however, it is decided, for alleged safety reasons, to reinforce with resin buildings built with other materials. At this point, the two-year experiment is ruined, and we will never know what the effect of the resin would have been compared to the other materials. If the buildings collapse, no one will know why. Perhaps the traditional material would have held up better and it was the resin that damaged it.

Neither ethics nor experimental science are slaves to law and political emergencies. Let's forget, therefore, the emergency authorization bureaucracy or its political criteria and ask ourselves the general problem raised by this breaking of the double blind. The substance of the matter is that there is, hypothetically, a phase of the experimental studies of drugs in which, albeit with partial results, it may become ethically required to break the double blind and give those who received the placebo the possibility of receiving the drug that we are testing. In reality, however, at the substantial level what we are talking about is a modification of the safety protocols of experimental science in a certain subject or area of research. The question, in fact, is whether an experiment shorter in time than initially foreseen is already able to provide appreciable results for the use of a certain drug. At stake, therefore, are not the ethical parameters of emergency authorization and double blinds, but the review of drug testing protocols which, hypothetically, should be attenuated or shortened.

The impression that a scholar like me has of the debate on breaking the double blind after emergency authorization decision is that someone wants to use it precisely for this reason, to lower the bar of experimental medical science and to change the safety protocols of drugs to business advantage of pharmaceutical companies. It is a fact that emergency authorizations are currently being treated as definitive, no longer seriously questioning their original parameters in light of developments and updates on efficacy and safety. Security protocols have indeed already changed. Is this what we wanted? Unfortunately, as I have said elsewhere, the current composition of the committees of the main relevant government agencies does not have the ethical and legal competence to scientifically address these issues.[115]

6.2.4. Admission of Guilt

The last aspect of this (somewhat mediocre) objection based on the large-scale administration of these new products is that of the admission of guilt that it implies on the part of those who agree with it, especially when it comes to people who have taken part in political choices and governmental policies regarding such products.

The question is simple. Let's take the logic of those who express that objection seriously. Covid vaccines are not *experimental*, so they say, because they have by now been tested on billions of people. But the alleged experimentation on these billions of people took place *after* the authorization to market, not before. If it is true that these vaccines are no longer experimental by virtue of this massive use following marketing, it logically follows that they were experimental at the time of marketing.

If this is the case, it means that these billions of people have tested a product in their bodies without having voluntarily consented to be part of a medical trial. This would naturally be a very serious violation of medical ethics and of the rules guaranteeing informed consent, as well as of the principle that no one can be subjected to human drug trials in a devious way and without consent.

Since the days of Nuremberg, it has been crystal clear that human experimentation cannot be conducted without consent that is actually free and verified, and also that it cannot be subtly promoted with misleading information and advertising—such as those already circulating on Covid vaccines for children to make them become knights in the fight against the virus or other nonsense of the kind. Of course, nothing is further from

115 See F. Di Blasi, *The Death of the Phronimos: Faith and Truth about Anti Covid Vaccines*, op. cit., chapter 2.3. "FDA and EMA."

the ethics of human experimentation than legal obligations, vaccine passports, public ostracism, and persecution. When people who belong to government agencies or to the governing bodies of a country say that Covid vaccines are not experimental because they have been used on billions of people, they are implicitly, but in a strong and evident way, admitting that they have used those same vaccines on billions of people violating all basic rules of medical ethics and human testing law.

The paradox is that those same people who insist on denying—against any scientific evidence, logical and epistemological criteria, and common-sense rules—that current vaccines are experimental do so precisely for this fear of being accused of having promoted (to the extent of compulsion) large-scale experiments on humans. Then, however, without realizing it and blinded by demagogy, they publicly use in support of the non-experimental nature of vaccines, an argument that implies their admission of guilt. This provides an additional sign, if needed, of the ethical and intellectual paucity of those who manage the fanatical propaganda on anti-Covid vaccines in this very sad period of our history.

6.3. The Importance of the Legal Aspect

The legal aspect of vaccines (supply contracts, emergency or conditional approvals, criminal shield or legal immunity, etc.) is fundamental for the purpose of moral choice also because the law has a technical advantage of truthfulness. In televised debates and in newspapers, everything is often said with great carelessness and aggression, people flippantly give more space to their personal opinions than to objective data, and they evaluate their statements on the basis of the audience. Unfortunately, even invited experts focus much more on their notoriety than on the information they give, and often base their tones and explanations on this non-scientific interest. When they appear on television, experts easily insult each other even in ways that would be unthinkable in academia or the professional world. Let's call it mass media disease, notoriety syndrome, or let's just call it human mediocrity. Let's call it what we want, but it remains an irrefutable fact: on television, we too often see the worst in people; we see a carousel of experts who speak with arrogance and superficiality about everything they are not experts in as if they were.

When law is involved, however, everything changes because law means responsibility. I remember once, in high school, that I went to the emergency room for a wound I had gotten from rusty pieces of iron. The doctor, in the presence of a couple of assistants and distracted by something else, told me that there was no need for a tetanus shot and that I could leave. I was not worried. I went to the hospital out of a general sense of responsibility, knowing the risk of tetanus. I replied, calmly and without discussing the merits of the matter in any way, that there was no problem, but that I wanted him to explain in writing that he felt it was unnecessary for me to receive a tetanus shot. Within seconds, a smile and the sting followed. From this, I, although still a high school student, was able to deduce that the doctor was not at all sure that tetanus medication was not necessary in my case, and that he would not have risked his professional responsibility. Since then, I have seen this same thing a million times in all professional fields: how certain a professional is of a matter that concerns his area of specialization can be seen from what he is willing to put in writing in a legal context.

The law has many defects but, at least, it also possesses this great virtue. It forces people to say exactly what they mean when signing a contract or writing a will. It forces experts to say exactly what they believe can be said about a certain issue when signing a report to be filed in court. For smart people, Europe's secret contracts with vaccine manufacturers were the first wake-up call. In those contracts (as we found out later) the pharmaceutical companies wrote exactly what they believed they could say with certainty: namely, that the vaccines were produced in rapid times dictated by the emergency, "*that the long-term effects and efficacy of the Vaccine are not currently known,*" that there could be negative effects and that purchasing governments must assume responsibility. If we add to these contracts the characteristics of emergency authorizations and other things such as American immunity and the Italian criminal shield, the objective framework of scientific certainties appears clearly. The rest is nonsense, games for TV talk shows and for poor and/or bad-faith politicians and journalists.

This discourse is obviously not against Covid vaccines, which people hope will eventually work, or at least that the benefits will outweigh the harms. It is against propaganda and against trivializations aimed at not making people think and preventing them from making decisions freely based on data and facts that are truly available, starting with the legal ones.

6.4. Vaccines Available in America and Europe

These two circumstances alone (i.e., the short-, medium-, and long-term unknowns and the emergency authorizations) already make it clear how much the choice to use these vaccines implies a delicate prudential reasoning that must take into account some technical unknowns. The use of these vaccines, in other words, is not a field in which one can have technical or moral certainties at the moment. Precisely for this reason, I do not tire of emphasizing it, there is a heightened ethical duty to correctly inform those who are to decide whether to use them (for themselves or for others). Giving false certainties is inherently irresponsible and ethically wrong.

This does not mean, of course, that an expert in any specific field related to the topic cannot be sure of his opinion on vaccines and cannot express it accordingly. However, it means that such an expert cannot hide from his public the objective uncertainties of the case also linked to the legal nature of the authorizations and to the different or contrary opinions of his colleagues. Furthermore, experts must always clarify the type of judgments they express (moral, legal, epidemiological, medical, virological, political, etc.), possibly issuing a warning when they leave their field of specialization and start talking about the issue as any ordinary person could do in dialogue with others and with their own moral conscience.

At the moment, there are three Covid vaccines available in the United States,

a. Comirnaty and Pfizer-BioNTech
b. Moderna
c. Janssen (Johnson & Johnson)

For these vaccines, the FDA reports, in specific documents and in a very clear way, both the technical data of the authorizations (with updates and chronological corrections) and FAQs and information sheets differentiated for those who must administer the vaccines and for those who must receive them. These factsheets are available in about thirty languages. It must be said, however, that the documents available in other languages are not usually updated. Some that I checked in Italian in September 2021 were still from December 2020 and there were no indications of the many adverse events that occurred thereafter. If a foreigner were to rely on those translations, he would face very serious misinformation. It is clear that the FDA, based on those documents in other languages, cares moreabout the political image of the appearance of a multilingual site than about people's health.[116]

In Europe, there are currently five licensed vaccines,

a. Comirnaty (Pfizer)
b. Spikevax (Moderna)
c. Janssen (Johnson & Johnson)
d. Vaxzevria (Oxford-AstraZeneca)

---

116 See FDA, "Covid-19 Vaccines," URL: https://www.fda.gov/emergency-preparedness-and-response/coronavirus-disease-2019-covid-19/covid-19-vaccines.

e. Nuvaxovid

For these vaccines, the EMA reports, in specific webpages (less clear than those of the FDA), a general presentation (overview), with questions and answers only in English, the details of the authorizations, information on the product and the history of evaluations and security updates. There is hardly anything available in other languages, not even the technical documents on the risk management plan. The comparison with the FDA (ignoring the unreliability of multilingual documents) is humiliating if you think that Europe, unlike the United States, is made up of countries which have their own national languages.[117]

All vaccines in use in Europe and the United States have also been recommended by the World Health Organization.[118]

117 See EMA, "Covid-19 vaccines," URL: https://www.ema.europa.eu/en/human-regulatory/overview/public-health-threats/coronavirus-disease-covid-19/treatments-vaccines/covid-19-vaccines.

118 See WHO (World Health Organization), "Covid-19 Vaccines," URL: https://www.who.int/emergencies/diseases/novel-coronavirus-2019/covid-19-vaccines - https://extranet.who.int/pqweb/sites/default/files/documents/Status_COVID_VAX_23Dec2021.pdf.

Chapter 7

The AstraZeneca Case: Decoy-rigged science and violation of informed consent

Nuvaxovid and AstraZeneca are the two anti-Covid vaccines with respect to which European developments take a different path from that of America. All the vaccines authorized in emergency mode by the FDA have in fact been approved (conditionally) also by the EMA for use in Europe. Indeed, there is almost always a correspondence between the decisions on the anti-Covid vaccines by the FDA and those by the EMA in the sense that the latter almost always follow those of the FDA by a couple of weeks, as if EMA tended in this area to align itself with the FDA. It could be mere coincidence. Or, as I tend to think, it could be due to the fact that the FDA has a capacity and financial base about twelve times larger than that of the EMA. The FDA has an annual budget of around six billion dollars versus around the five hundred million budget of the EMA.[119]

---

119 See my *The death of the Phronimos: Faith and Truth about anti-Covid Vaccines*, chap. 2. It should also be considered—as well highlighted by the transmission Report "In the hands of the vaccine" of January 25, 2021 based on the documents of Emaleaks—that the EMA received very strong political pressure and was accused precisely of not following the FDA's pace. It did not seem acceptable to politicians that the EMA

(continued on the next page)

Now, if we acknowledge that the FDA considers itself underpowered to face all its duties, to the point that it generally does not have sufficient staff to conduct inspections in the laboratories of pharmaceutical companies to directly view the drug testing phase, it can reasonably be inferred that all the more so the EMA is underpowered with respect to the processing of applications for authorization of anti-Covid vaccines. It can therefore be reasonably inferred that the EMA feels reassured in its decisions by following the FDA's prior work.

Two examples come to mind to illustrate this commonsense judgment. One concerns the recent case of FOIA access to the FDA records relating to Pfizer's approval.[120] The group of scholars who signed the FOIA symbolically gave the FDA 108 days to make the authorization documents available because this is the number of days that (supposedly) were sufficient for the FDA to evaluate the authorization of the vaccine. If in 108 days the FDA managed to study and evaluate the documentation of the application for approval, it is not clear why that timeframe should not be sufficient to make the application documents available to those who request them. Pfizer's submission, however, is an enormous dossier that is between 350,000 and 450,000 pages, or the equivalent of a library with more than two thousand books. The FDA then spontaneously proposed to the judge to be allowed to release five hundred pages a month, which would take between 55 and 75 years. Recently, the judge instead imposed on the FDA the delivery of 55,000 pages per month, responding to the FDA's objections of not having sufficient staff,

---

did not quickly approve in Europe what was approved in America by the FDA. The transmission of the Report in question is available at this URL: https://www.youtube.com/watch?v=-sf4r1GuLxI.

120 See F. Di Blasi, *The death of the Phronimos: Faith and Truth about anti-Covid Vaccines*, pp. 75-79.

that this transparency action, given the circumstances, must be a priority for the agency.[121]

The amount of work behind the approval of just one of these vaccines is truly impressive even compared to mere emergency authorizations. It is therefore surprising that the EMA has been able to process more applications than the FDA in record time, unless, in fact, the EMA is facilitated in its analysis, studies, and decisions by the previous decisions of the FDA. From this point of view, the evaluation of vaccines on which the FDA has not expressed itself assumes greater importance for the scholar, also from an ethical and epistemological point of view.

The other illustrative example I was thinking about was the recent Ventavia scandal, a large clinical research company used by Pfizer for some of their vaccine studies and tests. This scandal stems from revelations made to the *British Medical Journal*:

> "A regional director who was employed at the research organisation Ventavia Research Group has told *The BMJ* that the company falsified data, unblinded patients, employed inadequately trained vaccinators, and was slow to follow up on adverse events reported in Pfizer's pivotal phase III trial. Staff who conducted quality control checks were overwhelmed by the volume of problems they were finding. After repeatedly notifying Ventavia of these problems, the regional director, Brook Jackson, emailed a complaint to the US Food and Drug

121 See, e.g., J. Greene, "'Paramount importance': Judge orders FDA to hasten release of Pfizer vaccine docs," *Reuters*, January 7, 2022, URL: https://www.reuters.com/legal/government/paramount-importance-judge-orders-fda-hasten-release-pfizer-vaccine-docs-2022-01-07/?fbclid=IwAR0BQuQSZZMBhWQOQfe14kEG2jqtrJHLZZ1SIqXcnbpB1JAPUfGSkWN3kNA.

Administration (FDA). Ventavia fired her later the same day."[122]

The extent of this scandal is evident because it risks invalidating the very assumptions of the authorization granted by the FDA. Yet, despite the importance of the matter, the FDA, due to its alleged lack of personnel and resources, does not even seem to have made an inspection in the Ventavia Texan laboratories affected by the affair. I repeat, if the FDA claims to have such a lack of personnel that it is even prevented from carrying out control activities of this importance relating to American-made vaccines, what is the actual potential of the EMA to conduct an accurate examination on approvals in Europe of those same vaccines? If the FDA is having difficulty controlling laboratories in its country, what can the EMA do?

An in-depth study of vaccines approved only in Europe by the EMA can therefore also be interesting for us to see or evaluate EMA's accuracy and professionalism in cases where the FDA cannot lead the way. Nuvaxovid, however, is a new vaccine that received conditional approval from the EMA and emergency approval from the WHO only on December 20, 2021, and which has not yet finalized the application to the FDA for US emergency marketing authorization. AstraZeneca, on the other hand, has a much more interesting, complex, and *ancient* history (compared to the times of the pandemic), a history that also includes a missed American phase and that is an example of some important ethical and epistemological profiles that transversely concern all anti-Covid vaccines.

122 See P. D. Thacker, "Covid-19: Researcher blows the whistle on data integrity issues in Pfizer's vaccine trial," *British Medical Journal*, Published 02 November 2021, 375: n2635, doi:10.1136/bmj.n2635.

7.1. Non-Approval in the United States

Despite being one of the first Covid vaccines, AstraZeneca has never applied for emergency use authorization in the United States. The official technical reason (at least in the spring period) was that it preferred to first conclude phase 3 of its clinical trials as well as trials in the United States, since apparently the FDA, for purposes of its authorization, does not look kindly on clinical trials carried out abroad.

Some thought that AstraZeneca preferred at this point to ask for full approval directly instead of emergency use authorization. The story, however, is a bit more complex because there had already been a preliminary analysis for approval by the FDA Advisory Committee, but then the National Institutes of Health, headed by Anthony Fauci, accused AstraZeneca of including outdated data in their records. This was publicly acknowledged by AstraZeneca, which pledged to review the data within two days. By then however, a case had been created around the issue, generating an insurmountable public distrust of the vaccine (about which there were also other unclear data relating to clinical tests).[123] Add to this that, in March, there was a study in the *New England Journal of Medicine* that questioned the efficacy of

---

123 See, e.g., A. D. Sorkin, "Why There Is So Much Confusion About the AstraZeneca Vaccine," *The New Yorker*, March 23, 2021, URL: https://www.newyorker.com/news/daily-comment/why-there-is-so-much-confusion-about-the-astrazeneca-vaccine; T. Machemer, "Why U.S. Approval of the AstraZeneca Covid-19 Vaccine Is Taking So Long," *Smithsonian Magazine*, March 29, 2021, URL: https://www.smithsonianmag.com/smart-news/revised-astrazeneca-data-show-its-covid-19-vaccine-76-percent-effective-180977356/; M. Williams, "Why the US has not approved the AstraZeneca-Oxford Covid vaccine for use and is sending it abroad," *The Herald*, May 18, 2021, URL: https://www.heraldscotland.com/news/19310127.us-not-approved-astrazeneca-oxford-covid-vaccine-use-sending-abroad/.

AstraZeneca against variants,[124] and that there was a certain panic due to some cases of thrombosis about which the EMA also, in the same month, had expressed a very serious concern:

> "A causal link with the vaccine is not proven, but is possible and deserves further analysis."[125]

It must also be said that, at that point, the US market was already dominated by the other vaccines previously authorized, and AstraZeneca, even if authorized, would not have easily had access to an appreciable market share.

7.2. From Approval to Doubts

The doubts about the negative effects of the AstraZeneca vaccine were indeed very well founded. However, to understand their ethical importance we need to retrace the history of what happened in Europe, where the vaccine had in fact received

124 See S. A. Madhi, V. Baillie, C. L. Cutland, M. Voysey, A. L. Koen, L. Fairlie, F.C. Paeds., S. D. Padayachee, K. Dheda, S. L. Barnabas, Q. E. Bhorat, C. Briner, G. Kwatra, et al., for the NGS-SA Group, and the Wits-VIDA COVID Group, "Efficacy of the ChAdOx1 nCoV-19 Covid-19 Vaccine against the B.1.351 Variant," *The New England Journal of Medicine,* March 16, 2021, URL: https://www.nejm.org/doi/full/10.1056/NEJMoa2102214?query=featured_home.

125 See EMA, "COVID-19 Vaccine AstraZeneca: benefits still outweigh the risks despite possible link to rare blood clots with low blood platelets," News, March 18, 2021, URL: https://www.ema.europa.eu/en/news/covid-19-vaccine-astrazeneca-benefits-still-outweigh-risks-despite-possible-link-rare-blood-clots: "These are rare cases – around 20 million people in the UK and EEA had received the vaccine as of March 16 and EMA had reviewed only 7 cases of blood clots in multiple blood vessels (disseminated intravascular coagulation, DIC) and 18 cases of CVST. A causal link with the vaccine is not proven, but is possible and deserves further analysis."

emergency approval (called "conditional") in December 2020 in England—from the UK Medicines and Healthcare products Regulatory Agency (MHRA)—and on January 29, 2021, in the rest of Europe—by the EMA/EU Commission—for individuals aged 18 and over. It is interesting to retrace at least the salient features of this story because they reveal the ethical and epistemological attitude of some authorities involved towards these products subject to emergency/conditional authorizations.

It must be said that, at first, this vaccine seemed more suitable for the young or adult population than for the elderly, but this impression was perhaps due to the fact that almost all the pre-authorization studies had been conducted in the 18-55 age group. The elderly (few) were inserted only at a later time. I wonder if this initial target of the trials had been sufficiently evaluated given that Covid-19 was now notoriously an emergency disease only or above all with respect to the elderly and/or comorbid population.

Sometimes younger people are chosen for practical reasons independent from the adequacy of the experiment; for example, because it is easier to deal with people who do not have senile disorders or who do not need the consent of family members or guardians. According to this parameter, the choice of younger subjects is practical but erroneous compared to the emergency experimentation of a drug that has to fight a virus or a disease that mainly attacks the elderly population. Other times, unfortunately, the choice of younger subjects does not meet either scientific or ethical criteria, but only serves the distorted interests of the pharmaceutical industry. Young people or adults have stronger physiques that respond better to stress. Testing a new drug on younger subjects eliminates some potential negative side effects and in so doing, facilitates the drug's marketing.

In any case, on January 4, 2021, England launched a large-scale vaccination campaign starting (correctly) with the elderly and anticipating the use of the AstraZeneca vaccine by about a month compared to the rest of Europe. The European states, however, after a few weeks, already in the first part of March, began to suspend the use of the vaccine due to increasing reports of abnormal blood clotting. So did several countries around the world.[126] Worthy of note, in this context, is the declaration on March 15 by the Paul Ehrlich Institute—the German federal agency responsible for vaccines—that it had received

> "reports of cases of thrombotic events with concomitant thrombocytopenia in six women aged 20 to 49 years and one young man aged between 20-29 years who became symptomatic four to 16 days apart after receiving COVID-19 AstraZeneca vaccine. The six women developed central sinus vein thrombosis, two of which were fatal. A first observed versus expected analysis concluded that more cases of sinus thrombosis have been reported than would be expected by statistical chance."[127]

The British drug agency, on its own, declared that it was not confirmed that the blood clots were caused by the vaccine and that people could continue to be vaccinated.

> "Today the UK regulator, following a rigorous scientific review of all the available data, said that the available evidence does not suggest that blood clots in veins (venous

---

126 See, e.g., Al Jazeera News, "Which countries have stopped using AstraZeneca's COVID vaccine?," March 15, 2021, URL: https://www.aljazeera.com/news/2021/3/15/which-countries-have-halted-use-of-astrazenecas-covid-vaccine; J. Diaz, "Sweden, Venezuela Are Latest Countries To Question AstraZeneca Vaccine," NPR News, March 16, 2021, URL: https://www.npr.org/sections/coronavirus-live-updates/2021/03/16/977731757/sweden-venezuela-latest-countries-to-question-astrazeneca-vaccine.

127 See EMA, "Pharmacovigilance Risk Assessment Committee (PRAC)," April 8, 2021, URL: https://www.ema.europa.eu/en/documents/prac-recommendation/signal-assessment-report-embolic-thrombotic-events-smq-covid-19-vaccine-chadox1-s-recombinant_en.pdf.

thromboembolism) are caused by COVID-19 Vaccine AstraZeneca."[128]

"Following the rigorous scientific review, the MHRA concluded there is no evidence that blood clots in veins are occurring more than would be expected in the absence of vaccination."[129]

Even the WHO defended the vaccine in the first half of March by supporting a similar thesis, namely that hundreds of millions of doses of the vaccine have already been administered without any deaths being reported. This statement by the WHO is a slight example of erroneous or demagogic use of the sophism of a not-monitored synchronic intensity—that is, not detected or observed according to scientific parameters—as alleged evidence of the lack of adverse effects.[130]

In this first phase in England, there was a feeling that European countries were blocking the vaccine for a sort of post-Brexit revenge rather than for actual risks deriving from potential ad-

128 UK Government, "Government Response: UK regulator confirms that people should continue to receive the COVID-19 vaccine AstraZeneca," March 18, 2021, URL: https://www.gov.uk/government/news/uk-regulator-confirms-that-people-should-continue-to-receive-the-covid-19-vaccine-astrazeneca.

129 AstraZeneca, "UK and EU regulatory agencies confirm COVID-19 Vaccine AstraZeneca is safe and effective," March 18, 2021, URL: https://www.astrazeneca.com/media-centre/press-releases/2021/uk-and-eu-regulatory-agencies-confirm-covid-19-vaccine-astrazeneca-is-safe-and-effective.html.

130 See WHO, "WHO Director-General's opening remarks at the media briefing on COVID-19 – 12 March 2021," URL: https://www.who.int/director-general/speeches/detail/who-director-general-s-opening-remarks-at-the-media-briefing-on-covid-19-12-march-2021; Al Jazeera News, "WHO backs AstraZeneca coronavirus vaccine and plays down risks," March 12, 2021, URL: https://www.aljazeera.com/news/2021/3/12/who-backs-use-of-astrazeneca-vaccine-amid-blood-clot-fears.

verse effects encountered. There was probably some carelessness in the detection of adverse effects, of which the British drug agency seems to have received news since January, declaring, however, that it received the first reports only on February 8. A significant problem could also have arisen from having been cut off from the European pharmacovigilance system following Brexit.[131] On this exclusion from European pharmacovigilance, sooner or later a serious ethical legal debate should be opened, especially for similar emergency situations that could occur in the future.

7.3. The Turning Point of April 7

Il 7 aprile è una data tristemente importante per il vaccino Ast April 7 is a sadly important date for the AstraZeneca vaccine. First of all, a study by the Winton Center for Risk and Evidence

131 On these aspects, but also on the AstraZeneca case in general, see the excellent investigation of the Italian broadcast Report: in particular, the October 25, 2021 episode on the AstraZeneca vaccine, URL: https://www.raiplay.it/programmi/report. Report was one of the few examples of investigative journalism on the issue of vaccines in Italy which, however, recently (and contrary to expectations) has strangely given up on investigations on the subject. There is no doubt, from my point of view, that this is due to pressure from the governing parties. The public attack on Report, on the other hand, also by the other mainstream media subservient to the government was not a trivial matter. On the pro-government attitude of the mainstream media in Italy, a specific investigation should be carried out with respect to the public funds and funding received. In fact, these funds doubled in the pandemic phase, indicating a tendency of the government to buy the favor of the media, which has worked perfectly. See, e.g., S. Cannavò, "Il finanziamento pubblico ai giornali è raddoppiato," *Il Fatto Quotidiano*, December 29, 2021, URL: https://www.ilfattoquotidiano.it/in-edicola/articoli/2021/12/29/il-finanziamento-pubblico-ai-giornali-e-raddoppiato/6439851/.

Communication of the University of Cambridge was made public from which it emerged unequivocally that the risk-benefit ratio of the vaccine for the population under 30 was negative. In fact, in that age group, there was a non-existent risk of death from Covid compared to an actual risk of vaccine mortality. In general, it emerged that the benefits of the AstraZeneca vaccine tended to increase with age but gradually decreased from age 50 onwards.[132]

On the same day, an independent report from the British Government's Advisory Committee on Vaccination and Immunization (JCVI) was also released, recommending the use of a vaccine other than AstraZeneca, for ages 30 and under:

> "JCVI has weighed the relative balance of benefits and risks and advise that the benefits of prompt vaccination with the AstraZeneca COVID-19 vaccine far outweigh the risk of adverse events for individuals 30 years of age and over and those who have underlying health conditions which put them at higher risk of severe COVID-19 disease. JCVI currently advises that it is preferable for adults aged <30 years without underlying health conditions that put them at higher risk of severe COVID-19 disease, to be offered an alternative COVID-19 vaccine, if available. People may make an informed choice to receive the AstraZeneca COVID-19 vaccine to receive earlier protection."[133]

---

132 See Winton Centre for Risk and Evidence Communication, "News - Communicating the potential benefits and harms of the AstraZeneca COVID-19 vaccine," April 7, 2021, URL: https://wintoncentre.maths.cam.ac.uk/news/communicating-potential-benefits-and-harms-astra-zeneca-covid-19-vaccine/.

133 See UK Department of Health & Social Care, "Independent Report: JCVI statement on use of the AstraZeneca COVID-19 vaccine," April 7, 2021, URL: https://www.gov.uk/government/publications/use-of-the-astrazeneca-

(continued on the next page)

On the same day, the British Medicines Agency (MHRA), while not formally recommending any age restrictions in the use of the AstraZeneca vaccine,[134] accounted for the possible connection with blood clots, accounted for the JCVI judgment, and initiated a government's public change of course on the use of the vaccine, which would no longer be recommended for those under 30 years of age. The decision was announced in all the newspapers.[135]

For my purposes, it is important to stress that the change in the risk-benefit ratio for the younger age group compared to the older ones was not a subtlety limited to discussions between experts, but immediately reached the general public also through the news. The inversion of the benefit-risk ratio is the reason why the British public authorities, while continuing to emphasize the general benefits of the vaccine, changed the public indications

---

covid-19-vaccine-jcvi-statement/jcvi-statement-on-use-of-the-astrazeneca-covid-19-vaccine-7-april-2021.

134 "The MHRA is not recommending age restrictions in COVID-19 Vaccine AstraZeneca vaccine use": See UK Government, "Press Release: MHRA issues new advice, concluding a possible link between COVID-19 Vaccine AstraZeneca and extremely rare, unlikely to occur blood clots," April 7, 2021, URL: https://www.gov.uk/government/news/mhra-issues-new-advice-concluding-a-possible-link-between-covid-19-vaccine-astrazeneca-and-extremely-rare-unlikely-to-occur-blood-clots.

135 See, e.g., N. Triggle, "Covid: Under-30s offered alternative to Oxford-AstraZeneca jab," BBC News, April 7, 2021, URL: https://www.bbc.com/news/health-56665517; M. Cheng, D. Kirka, J. Lawless, "UK advises limiting AstraZeneca in under-30s amid clot worry," AP News, April 8, 2021, URL: https://apnews.com/article/eu-rare-blood-clots-possibly-linked-astrazeneca-vaccine-1ec87a9b7f14f98e29962e9d055d27ed.

for age groups, also with the aim of protecting the informed consent of citizens.[136]

7.4. The EMA's Immoral Turn-Around

On April 23, 2021, the EMA presented the results of the updated studies on the safety of the AstraZeneca vaccine at a press conference.[137] These studies were based above all on the collaboration with the Winton Center for Risk and Evidence Communication of Cambdrige, from whose study of April 7 they took the same graphs and tables and which they officially recognized in the concluding acknowledgements.[138]

On the same day, April 23, in addition to the streaming press conference, the EMA also issued a detailed press release accompanied by bibliographical information.[139] In this information, however, there is no reference to the study of the Winton Center for Risk and Evidence Communication, even if the EMA update technical document that I have just cited is

136 On this it is enough to see the ITV News of April 7, 2021: see T. Clarke, "Covid: Under 30s won't be given AstraZeneca vaccine over 'extremely rare' risk of blood clots," ITV News, April 7, 2021, URL: https://www.itv.com/news/2021-04-07/covid-oxford-vaccine-astrazeneca-press-briefing-jcvi-mhra.

137 See EMA, "Press briefing to update on analysis of data on Vaxzevria, the COVID-19 vaccine from AstraZeneca," April 23, 2021, URL: https://www.ema.europa.eu/en/events/ema-press-briefing-update-analysis-data-vaxzevria-covid-19-vaccine-astrazeneca.

138 See EMA, "Annex to Vaxzevria Art.5.3 - Visual risk contextualization," April 23, 2021, URL: https://www.ema.europa.eu/en/documents/chmp-annex/annex-vaxzevria-art53-visual-risk-contextualisation_en.pdf.

139 See EMA News, "AstraZeneca's COVID-19 vaccine: benefits and risks in context," April 23, 2021, URL: https://www.ema.europa.eu/en/news/astrazenecas-covid-19-vaccine-benefits-risks-context.

based almost entirely upon it. Instead, two scientific studies appear: one concerning people respectively from 70 years upwards and from 80 years upwards,[140] and the other, from February 19 (and therefore relating to a period that preceded the March emergency and shortly followed the start of vaccine use in Europe), relating to the reduction of hospitalizations in Scotland.[141] The collaboration with the Winton Center for Risk and Evidence Communication and its April 7 study did not appear in the press conference or in the press release. Only those who take the trouble to look for the EMA's technical annex know about them.

These two facts - that is, the concealment of the Winton Center for Risk and Evidence Communication and the bibliographic references of the press release (which have nothing to do

140 J. L. Bernal, N. Andrews, C. Gower, J. Stowe, C. Robertson, E. Tessier, R. Simmons, S. Cottrell, R. Roberts, M. O'Doherty, K. Brown, C. Cameron, D. Stockton, J. McMenamin, M. Ramsay, "Early effectiveness of COVID-19 vaccination with BNT162b2 mRNA vaccine and ChAdOx1 adenovirus vector vaccine on symptomatic disease, hospitalisations and mortality in older adults in England," *medRxiv*, March 3, 2021, 21252652; doi: https://doi.org/10.1101/2021.03.01.21252652.

141 E. Vasileiou, C. R. Simpson, C. Robertson, et al., "Effectiveness of First Dose of COVID-19 Vaccines Against Hospital Admissions in Scotland: National Prospective Cohort Study of 5.4 Million People," Preprints with *The Lancet*, Posted: February 19, 2021, Available at SSRN: https://ssrn.com/abstract=3789264 or http://dx.doi.org/10.2139/ssrn.3789264. I want to emphasize again that, while in England the use of the vaccine started on January 4, in the rest of Europe it started only in February, after the authorization of the EMA at the end of January. This study, therefore, cannot reasonably be of help to any serious and reliable European evaluation regarding the vaccine in question. The mere fact of mentioning it with respect to a European update at the end of April on the overall risk-benefit assessment appears negligent and in bad faith.

with the technical emergency in March) - already made it possible for any careful scholar to predict that the EMA was preparing to make decisions that were not in line with at least some of the main evidence from the Winton Center study. Let's see if that was true.

What did the EMA tell us on April 23, 2021? The press release summarized what was said at the press conference by EMA's Deputy Executive Director, Noël Wathion, and by the EMA Head of Analytics, Peter Harlett, who focused in particular on the methodology of analysis. The crux of the matter is that

> "The benefits of Vaxzevria outweigh its risks in adults of all age groups; however, very rare cases of blood clots with low blood platelets have occurred following vaccination."[142]

The press release also explained that the EMA Medical Committee (CHMP) analyzed the benefits and risks of "unusual blood clots with low platelets" in different age groups, adding that

> "The analysis looked at prevention of hospitalisations, ICU admissions and deaths due to COVID-19, based on different assumptions of vaccine effectiveness to contextualise the occurrence of these unusual blood clots. It showed that the benefits of vaccination increase with increasing age and infection rates."[143]

However, nothing was said about the decrease in benefits with decreasing age, especially with reference to the groups under 30. Harlett explained that the risks and benefits are calculated according to three levels of risk exposure (high, medium, and low) and with respect to the three parameters of hospitalizations, intensive care, and deaths. The most surprising thing is that, with respect to the sources and data used, the press release

142 See EMA News, "AstraZeneca's COVID-19 vaccine: benefits and risks in context," op. cit.
143 Ibid.

made a generic reference to the European Center for Disease Prevention and Control, to the contribution of the member states, and to the Eudravigilance system (for pharmacovigilance), but then added that "it then determined the number of events the vaccine would prevent" using the data from the two "observational studies" I mentioned above, namely, the one on the elderly over 70 and 80 years old and the one in February on hospitalizations in Scotland, which are not in themselves adquate to justify the conclusions of the EMA. There is no mention of the Winton Center—the only one, I repeat, with specific data for the age groups at risk (and which is thanked in the annex).

Or rather, there is a trace of a mention, but you have to know how to recognize it. Harlett, in fact, in support of his explanation states that "nine graphs have been published today" to summarize the EMA's conclusions on the benefits of the vaccine.[144] But these nine graphs are simply the reworking of those taken from the Winton Center (with a lot of thanks) - those same graphs that had caused the turning point of April 7 in England. The only difference is that the Winton Center had made three graphs, divided according to risk levels (high, medium, and low) but with aggregated data with respect to hospitalizations, intensive care, and death, while the EMA disaggregated them into nine graphs (making three for each of the three events).

7.4.1. Eccentric Assessments of Risks and Benefits

The EMA's April 23 assessment that vaccine benefits outweigh risks in all age groups did not go completely unnoticed. I remember that when I listened to the reports of Wathion and Harlett at the press conference, I was in a hurry to devote myself to something else, but I thought it was impossible that the journalists present would not express any doubts about it. I then con-

144 These graphs are naturally those of the annex. See EMA, "Annex to Vaxzevria Art.5.3 - Visual risk contextualization," already cited.

tinued to listen to the entire question and answer session, waiting impatiently for the topic to come up.

When the questions began, Harlett was on the defensive. He evaded the first questions by claiming that he was not there to give numbers, but instead to invite us to contextualize the benefits of the vaccine in the overall scenarios that emerged from the nine graphs. Marco Cavaleri, Head of the Anti-Infectives and Vaccines, Scientific and Regulatory Management Department at the EMA, who was present but had not reported, said, in response to a question, that the causes of the blood clots were unknown. I report this detail not because it is necessary for my current ethical discourse, but only as an example of what I explained earlier on the epistemology of epidemiology and pharmacovigilance. Statistical science that leads to prudence-based decisions on Covid vaccines does not express the why of things and can be defined as experimental science only in a very diluted and limited sense of the term. The EMA did not give the data on the AstraZeneca vaccine because it knew the reason for the adverse effects, or because it really knew the *science*.

But let's go back to the press conference, which proceeded in a rather boring way with the speakers basically repeating things already said before. That was at least until it came to Susie Ardai, from Bloomberg, whom I thank for rewarding my patience. Susie asked why the recommendation for the under 30 age group, and perhaps even the under 40 group, hadn't changed, as the graphs looked like the risks outweighed the benefits. Harlett replied that if you looked at just one isolated benefit, then Susie's doubt was well founded, but if you looked at the overall picture of all benefits over all scenarios, things changed. If one considered that in some member countries, there was a high level of infection, he added, then one would understand that the risk-benefit balance remained positive in all scenarios.

Let's analyze what Harlett said with respect to the various scenarios for the under 30 age group. After all, these are extremely simple charts. First, however, a note regarding Harlett is a must.

His answer has this logical structure: 1) compared to the single isolated benefit Susie would be right, 2) but we have to look at all the benefits and all the scenarios, 3) considering that some countries have a high level of contagion. Point 3) of Harlett's, however, concerns only one of the scenarios, the one with a high risk of contagion. Logically, it should therefore be equated with Harlett's objection to Susie in point 1), that is, the (alleged) error of looking at a single datum isolated from the others. Harlett criticizes Susie because by hypothesis, she focuses on only one benefit (although it is not clear what it is according to Harlett), but his answer is also based on a single scenario, that of some member states with a high level of contagion. These contradictions are typical of those who flounder a little, to put it humorously. Now let's see why Harlett was fumbling and why he basically faced a press conference without ever accepting a real debate.

7.4.2. The Proper Weight of Death, Intensive Care, and Hospitalizations

Before analytically reviewing the details of the individual scenarios, however, I must draw attention to a fundamental ethical error in the EMA's decision of April 23. The logic of this decision is based (albeit in a way that has yet to be verified) on shifting attention from the risk of death to the benefits of the vaccine also with respect to hospitalizations and intensive care. But does it make sense to put these three things on the same level with respect to the risk-benefit assessment? From what point of view is such a choice made? How many hospitalizations does one death equal?

There is no doubt that neither medical nor statistical science can express preferences or assessments between death events, intensive care, and hospitalization. A utilitarian politician might perhaps say that he prefers one death to a hundred hospitalizations because the latter cost the legal system so much. The inhumanity of such a statement is obvious, but this is not what I am interested in highlighting. I just want to clarify that the evaluative choice between a risk of death and a risk of hospitalization cannot fall within the competence of the sciences which Wathion and Harlett express. Deaths and hospitalizations are similar in numbers, or quantity, but heterogeneous in substance, or quality. To be precise, the only sciences that could have a say on whether, under certain conditions, to prefer the risk of death to the risk of hospitalization are ethics and anthropology, or even theology, but certainly not medicine or statistics. On the basis of what medical tools and concepts could a patient be told, for example, that it is better for him, in general, to risk losing a leg rather than an arm or vice versa?

Here the epistemological problem is significant. If Wathion and Harlett say they have done the benefit-risk assessment by numerically comparing the risks of death, intensive care, and hospitalization, they complete an illogical operation that contradicts their science. The only scientific data that they can express is the numerical one of how many deaths, hospitalizations, or intensive care are risked in certain cases, but the qualitative comparison between these events for the purposes of the overall risk-benefit assessment is not their responsibility. This overall assessment, if anything, must be left clearly to those who have to decide for themselves on the vaccine. Making the public believe that they possess a science capable of expressing the overall benefit-risk assessment of those heterogeneous events is not only a scientific but an ethical error. It amounts to deception and to a violation of informed consent.

7.4.3. The Importance of the Contagion Risk Factor and of Personal Behavior

Another scientific clarification to be made in general concerns high, medium, and low risk factors. Harlett suggests that the analysis and assessment of these risk factors is a fact that he already possesses and that can be applied to individual countries and, ultimately, to his overall assessment of the entire European territory. In fact, this is what he does at the press conference: he says that, in light of the high-risk factor of some European states, it can be said that the benefits of the vaccine always outweigh the risks regardless of age groups.

This claim is scientifically erroneous for several reasons. I have already highlighted one. If Harlett's assessment is based on all possible scenarios, his conclusion cannot be determined by a single scenario. Another mistake is geographical. If one country is high-risk and another low-risk, there is no scientific criterion for recommending the vaccine to citizens of the two states in the same way. There is certainly no statistical criterion that legitimizes such a conclusion. Harlett does not have a science that can compare or equate two states with different scenarios. Again, Harlett's evaluative conclusions are not in harmony with his statistical premises.

There is another much more important issue that I wanted to point out, however, and which relates to informed consent. A high, medium, or low risk factor cannot only be considered abstractly on large numbers. This is a scientifically limited type of generalization whose limitations cannot be ignored by people who have to make vital decisions regarding their health and a possible risk of their own death.

Let's assume, for example, that a certain state statistically has a high contagion risk. This statistical data on large numbers, however, says almost nothing to those who, in that state, live for example in the countryside or in an isolated mountain town with very few contacts with the metropolises. If I am in a low-risk individual situation, what I expect from statistical science is that it will tell me the numbers of the low-risk scenario so that I can adjust accordingly. If anything, I expect epidemiological medical science to clarify the behavioral models capable of exposing me to greater or lesser risks. Still, I could live in a high-risk city but decide to adopt extremely restrictive behavior models that make me fall within the parameters of a medium or low risk scenario. Again, what I need from statistical science is not a generalizing erroneous judgment, but concrete numbers of the risks of the real individual scenarios.

A fair informed consent precisely presupposes this: to clarify to people what the risk factors are so that everyone can modify his behaviors and decisions accordingly. Here again, the scientist does not have to make assessments for me based on generalizations that potentially do not fit my case. These assessments are wrong, or are correct only if they make more accurate references, saying, for example: "Keep in mind that, in general, there is this level of risk in this territory and that, consequently, if you are not in situations that distinguish you from the average of the territory or if you do not adopt particular levels of personal precaution, the evaluation of the risks and benefits of the vaccine is this for hospitalizations, this for intensive care, and this for death." The scientist who does not clarify these epistemological limits and suggests that there is a single risk-benefit assessment and a single piece of advice to be given in this regard is making, here too, both a scientific error and an ethical error, with a very serious violation of informed consent.

7.4.4. The Three Scenarios of Informed Consent

Let's now look at the nine scenarios of the EMA technical document cited by Harlett. For simplicity's sake and to stay on the subject, I will reference the parameters for people under 30 in each scenario. All scenario data should be read on a 100,000-person basis after the first dose.

a. High contagion risk

I. Hospitalisations

Age	Cases of COVID-19 Hospitalisations prevented	Cases of blood clots with low platelets
20-29	64	1.9
30-39	81	1.8
40-49	122	2.1
50-59	208	1.1
60-69	324	1
70-79	547	0.5
80+	1239	0.4

- Potential benefits under 30: 64 prevented hospitalizations
- Potential harm under 30: 1.9 cases of blood clots with low platelets

II. ICU

Age	Cases of COVID-19 ICU admissions prevented	Cases of blood clots with low platelets
20-29	6	1.9
30-39	8	1.8
40-49	15	2.1
50-59	28	1.1
60-69	50	1
70-79	78	0.5
80+	110	0.4

- Potential benefits under 30: 6 prevented intensive therapies
- Potential harm under 30: 1.9 cases of blood clots with low platelets

III. Death

Age	Cases of COVID-19 deaths prevented	Cases of blood clots with low platelets
20-29	0	1.9
30-39	3	1.8
40-49	10	2.1
50-59	14	1.1
60-69	45	1
70-79	172	0.5
80+	733	0.4

- Potential benefits under 30: 0 deaths prevented
- Potential harm under 30: 1.9 cases of blood clots with low platelets

b. Medium Contagion risk

I. Hospidalisation

Age	Cases of COVID-19 Hospitalisations prevented	Cases of blood clots with low platelets
20-29	37	1.9
30-39	54	1.8
40-49	81	2.1
50-59	114	1.1
60-69	183	1
70-79	278	0.5
80+	332	0.4

- Potential benefits under 30: 37 prevented hospitalizations
- Potential harm under 30: 1.9 cases of blood clots with low platelets

II. ICU

Age	Cases of COVID-19 ICU admissions prevented	Cases of blood clots with low platelets
20-29	3	1.9
30-39	5	1.8
40-49	10	2.1
50-59	15	1.1
60-69	28	1
70-79	39	0.5
80+	29	0.4

- Potential benefits under 30: 3 prevented intensive therapies
- Potential harm under 30: 1.9 cases of blood clots with low platelets

III. Death

Age	Cases of COVID-19 deaths prevented	Cases of blood clots with low platelets
20-29	0	1.9
30-39	2	1.8
40-49	7	2.1
50-59	8	1.1
60-69	25	1
70-79	87	0.5
80+	197	0.4

- Potential benefits under 30: 0 deaths prevented
- Potential harm under 30: 1.9 cases of blood clots with low platelets

c. Low Contagion risk

I. Hospedalisations

Age	Cases of COVID-19 Hospitalisations prevented	Cases of blood clots with low platelets
20-29	4	1.9
30-39	5	1.8
40-49	6	2.1
50-59	10	1.1
60-69	19	1
70-79	45	0.5
80+	151	0.4

- Potential benefits under 30: 4 prevented hospitalizations
- Potential harm under 30: 1.9 cases of blood clots with low platelets

II. ICU

Age	Cases of COVID-19 ICU admissions prevented	Cases of blood clots with low platelets
20-29	0	1.9
30-39	0	1.8
40-49	1	2.1
50-59	1	1.1

60-69	3	1
70-79	6	0.5
80+	13	0.4

- Potential benefits under 30: 0 prevented intensive care
- Potential harm under 30: 1.9 cases of blood clots with low platelets

III. Death

Age	Cases of COVID-19 deaths prevented	Cases of blood clots with low platelets
20-29	0	1.9
30-39	0	1.8
40-49	1	2.1
50-59	1	1.1
60-69	3	1
70-79	14	0.5
80+	90	0.4

- Potential benefits under 30: 0 deaths prevented
- Potential harm under 30: 1.9 cases of blood clots with low platelets

A person aged 30 or under who is confronted with this scientific data for the purposes of his informed consent to the vaccine immediately notices that there is no scenario in which the vaccine offers the benefit of preventing Covid deaths. However, he notes that all three events of death, intensive care, and hospitalizations are contrasted with a generic risk of about two cases of blood clots with low platelets, which means that there is an aggregate risk that can imply death (as indeed already emerged from the Paul Ehrlich Institute data and as sadly happened after April to a greater extent). In preventing death, therefore, the administration of the vaccine generates only a risk without providing any benefit.

In preventing treatment in intensive care units, the benefit is practically nil in the medium and low risk scenarios and minimal in the high-risk scenario, in which 6 intensive therapies are avoided for every hundred thousand vaccine administrations: this is a decidedly insignificant percentage. Hospitalizations are the only case that presents a (albeit statistically insignificant) difference in the high and medium risk scenarios compared to low risk. Those who do not take the vaccine risk being one of 64 (high risk) or 37 (low risk) people who, for every 100,000 doses, will end up taking a trip to the hospital.

It is quite clear that if I (for whatever reason) found myself in a low-risk scenario, I would have absolutely no benefit from taking the vaccine, but would instead run a (albeit minimal) risk of death. No sane person would choose to be vaccinated under these conditions. If I were in a medium-risk scenario, I would have to ask myself if 37 potential hospitalizations are preferable to two deaths—an assessment which of course has no statistical nature. Again, I don't think any sane person would choose to take a vaccine that could cause death just to avoid a minimal risk of ending up in the hospital for a few days. Even in the high-risk scenario, however, and with all due respect to Harlett, no sane person would choose the vaccine. In fact, even in this scenario, the risk of ending up in hospital is not qualitatively comparable to the risk of death.

Let's now look at the purely numerical data of all the scenarios, as if the risks and events were all on the same level. Harlett is certainly right here. Five out of nine scenarios show benefits outweighing the potential harms. And even considering the overall numbers (aggregating all the scenarios and putting benefits on one side and risks on the other), those of hospitalizations alone exceed any other number.

However, if we look, even from a purely numerical point of view, at the statistical significance of the scenarios, it is already difficult to agree with Harlett even from the purely quantitative point of view of his *science*. The numbers of high- and medium-risk ICUs and low-risk hospitalizations are, in fact, too close to the potential harm to generate a truly significant difference. With respect to the evaluation of the decision to vaccinate or not (even limited to the purely quantitative data), it would be better to consider them as irrelevant scenarios and exclude them. In other words, if someone for example told me that the vaccine, every 100,000 doses, has a potential benefit of 3 (average risk) and a harm of 1.9, I would reasonably conclude that these are not relevant differences. If we exclude these scenarios with too close numbers, however, the only scenarios in which the benefits statistically significantly outweigh the risks remain two out of nine: that is, the scenarios of higher numbers of potentially avoided hospitalizations in high- and medium-risk circumstances. Ultimately, if we look at the numerical data in this way, the EMA's (and Harlett's) judgment on the risk-benefit assessment of the vaccine appears ridiculous and scientifically unfounded even from a quantitative or statistical point of view.

If we then break the quantitative numerical mold, so to speak, and look at the substance of the risks and benefits, the very idea that two scenarios in which some hospitalizations are potentially spared justify the positive judgment on a vaccine that can cause death appears grotesque and scandalous. I can't imagine how any intelligent person or person with a shred of morality can come up with this thesis. Admitted and not granted, however, that the EMA officials think such a judgment is possible, hiding the disaggregated data from citizens by making them believe there is a single exact and scientific assessment of the risks and benefits of that data remains an inadmissible violation of informed consent. It remains something that someone should answer for, given the deaths that followed this decision. I believe that the EMA, on this specific issue and for transparency, should open an internal investigation or disciplinary proceedings to ascertain what actually happened.

In a state like Italy, for example, based mainly on the EMA data from April 23, the AstraZeneca vaccine continued to be recommended to everyone without distinction of age groups, even promoting days of mass vaccination up to the month of June.[145] The error was also facilitated by the fact that the Italian Medicines Agency (AIFA) reported the adverse effects in an aggregate way, showing only one serious case in a million cases, whereas the cases of thrombosis with low platelets for women under the age of 60 ranged from two to four for every hundred thousand doses.[146] It seems that the European pharmacovigilance data were also ignored, which gave more or less one serious case for every ten thousand vaccinations. This madness based on a mixture of ignorance and disinformation stopped only with the death of an eighteen-year-old girl, Camilla Canepa, one of the victims of this collective ignorance and fanaticism.[147]

I frankly wonder if it is really possible that all the experts of the Government Scientific Technical Committee (CTS) and of the Italian government agencies ignored without gross negligence the falsified data and advice that was presented by the EMA on April 23. Would it have been so difficult to check the bibliography and the technical annex? On this too we will have to wait for some

---

145 See Italian Government, Comitato Tecnico Scientifico (Scientific Technical Committee - CTS), meeting minutes no. 17 of May 12, 2021, URL: https://emergenze.protezionecivile.gov.it/it/sanitarie/coronavirus/verbali-comitato-tecnico-scientifico.

146 See AIFA, "Covid vaccine surveillance report 19 - period December 27, 2020-September 26, 2021," n. 9, URL: https://www.aifa.gov.it/documents/20142/1315190/Rapporto_sorveglianza_vaccini_COVID-19_9.pdf.

147 On the detailed reconstruction of these events, see Report, episode of October 25, 2021, already mentioned.

diligent magistrate to take action after the collective psychosis has passed.

Apart from the case of subjects under 30—which I specifically focused on because that was what the English recommendation of April 7 saw in direct contrast to those of the EMA of April 23—I invite readers to try to make their own personal assessment of risks and benefits based on those nine scenarios also with respect to other age groups. For the purposes of this assessment, of course, one must also consider that the vaccine presents unknown risks, while the scenarios indicate only the currently foreseeable damage. From this point of view, I believe that it is logically impossible to conclude that the vaccine can be a sensible choice even under the age of 40 and that it is very unlikely to consider it sensible even under the age of 50 or 60. If a person who falls within these age groups, for example, by virtue of one's personal precautions and the geographic or logistical condition in which he lives, looks roughly at medium and low risk scenarios, the foreseeable advantages of the vaccine do not appear in any way significant, especially when the unpredictable risks are added to the picture. Still, I am not interested in making these assessments for others. It is enough that everyone can observe these data that the EMA had available and make their own informed decision— which is the very thing that the EMA wanted to prevent.

Chapter 8

Final Pfizer Approval by the FDA

It is an important fact that only one Covid vaccine has been given full authorization for individuals over the age of 16 at the moment, as of August 23, 2021 and by a single agency (the American FDA).[148] For subjects in the age group 12-15, the emergency authorization was renewed on the same day, while the extension of the emergency authorization of the primary dose of the vaccine to younger subjects in the age group 5-11 was given on October 29, 2021.[149]

Let me recall that in this text my objective is not the analysis of the specific application circumstances of the anti-Covid vaccines, but the analysis of the structural institutional circumstances. The specific issues of some Covid vaccines are relevant here as they highlight or exemplify the general epistemological and ethical problems of authorizations and consequent marketing.

148 See FDA News Release, "FDA Approves First COVID-19 Vaccine," August 23, 2021, URL: https://www.fda.gov/news-events/press-announcements/fda-approves-first-covid-19-vaccine.

149 See FDA, "Comirnaty and Pfizer-BioNTech COVID-19 Vaccine," URL: https://www.fda.gov/emergency-preparedness-and-response/coronavirus-disease-2019-covid-19/comirnaty-and-pfizer-biontech-covid-19-vaccine.

8.1. Criticism in the British Medical Journal (BMJ)

Pfizer's definitive authorization has been strongly criticized by leading voices in the scientific world for its haste, politicalization, and lack of transparency. In this regard, the immediate and very strong position of the British Medical Journal is worth reading.

> "COVID-19: FDA SET TO GRANT FULL APPROVAL TO PFIZER VACCINE WITHOUT PUBLIC DISCUSSION OF DATA.
>
> Transparency advocates have criticised the US Food and Drug Administration's (FDA) decision not to hold a formal advisory committee meeting to discuss Pfizer's application for full approval of its Covid-19 vaccine. Last year the FDA said it was "committed to use an advisory committee composed of independent experts to ensure deliberations about authorisation or licensure are transparent for the public. But in a statement, the FDA told *The BMJ* that it did not believe a meeting was necessary ahead of the expected granting of full approval. [...] The vaccine has already been rolled out to millions of Americans through an emergency use authorisation. Companies typically apply for full approval after a longer period has elapsed so that more data are available for review. But with the US government indicating this week that it plans to start making booster shots widely available next month, experts said the decision not to meet to discuss the data was politically driven.
>
> DATA SCRUTINY
>
> Kim Witczak, a drug safety advocate who serves as a consumer representative on the FDA's Psychopharmacologic Drugs Advisory Committee, said the decision removed an important mechanism for scrutinising the data.
>
> "These public meetings are imperative in building trust and confidence especially when the vaccines came to

market at lightning speed under emergency use authorisation," she said. "The public deserves a transparent process, especially as the call for boosters and mandates are rapidly increasing. These meetings offer a platform where questions can be raised, problems tackled, and data scrutinised in advance of an approval."

Witczak is one of the more than 30 signatories of a citizen petition calling on the FDA to refrain from fully approving any Covid-19 vaccine this year to gather more data. She warned that without a meeting "we have no idea what the data looks like."

"It is already concerning that full approval is being based on 6 months' worth of data despite the clinical trials designed for two years," she said. "There is no control group after Pfizer offered the product to placebo participants before the trials were completed.

"Full approval of Covid-19 vaccines must be done in an open public forum for all to see. It could set a precedent of lowered standards for future vaccine approvals."

PUBLIC DISCUSSION

Diana Zuckerman, president of the National Center for Health Research, who has also spoken at recent VRBPAC meetings, told *The BMJ*, "It's obvious that the FDA has no intention of hearing anyone else's opinion. But if you make decisions behind closed doors it can feed into hesitancy. It's important to have a public discussion about what kind of data are there and what the limitations are. As we think about risk versus benefit, we need to know."

Joshua Sharfstein, vice dean for public health practice and community engagement at the Johns Hopkins Bloomberg School of Public Health and former FDA deputy commissioner during the Obama administration, said that advisory committee meetings were more than just a way of receiving scientific input from outside ex-

> perts. "It's also an opportunity to educate the public about the important work that the FDA has done reviewing an enormous amount of data about a product," he told *The BMJ.* "It's a chance for questions to be asked and answered, building public confidence.
>
> "If there are no advisory committee meetings prior to licensure, the FDA should consider taking extra steps to explain the basis of its decisions to the public."
>
> On 18 August, before the news that the FDA would not be holding a formal committee meeting, the president of the Infectious Diseases Society of America Barbara Alexander praised the impact of the VRBPAC meetings as "a critical and necessary part" of the process for assessing whether to give booster doses."[150]

This note from the BMJ is supported by an article by one of the senior editors of the journal, Peter Doshi, professor of pharmaceutical health services research, whose field of specialization concerns precisely the process of approval of drugs, the way in which risks and benefits of medical products are assessed and communicated, and how to improve the credibility and accuracy of the evidence synthesis and biomedical publications.[151]

---

150 See *British Medical Journal*, "*Covid-19: FDA set to grant full approval to Pfizer vaccine without public discussion of data*," August 20, 2021, URL: https://www.bmj.com/content/374/bmj.n2086?fbclid=IwAR3VGq5roC6ZVs-H7rgaInYA4DNoDgq-SmwJAVMhM6znSVP0zdJ8W__VzcU. The emphasis is mine.

151 See P. Doshi's profile on the BMJ, https://www.bmj.com/about-bmj/editorial-staff/peter-doshi: "Peter Doshi is a senior editor at The BMJ and on the News & Views team. Based in Baltimore, he is also an associate professor of pharmaceutical health services research at the University of Maryland School of Pharmacy. His research focuses on the drug approval process, how the risks and benefits of medical products are assessed and communicated, and improving the credibility and accuracy of evidence synthesis and biomedical publications."

"[...] Last December, with limited data, the FDA granted Pfizer's vaccine an EUA, enabling access to all Americans who wanted one. It sent a clear message that the FDA could both address the enormous demand for vaccines without compromising on the science. A "full approval" could remain a high bar.

But here we are, with FDA reportedly on the verge of granting a marketing license 13 months into the still ongoing, two year pivotal trial, with no reported data past 13 March 2021, unclear efficacy after six months due to unblinding,[152] evidence of waning protection irrespective of the Delta variant, and limited reporting of safety data. (The preprint reports "decreased appetite, lethargy, asthenia, malaise, night sweats, and hyperhidrosis were new adverse events attributable to BNT162b2 not previously identified in earlier reports," but provides no data tables showing the frequency of these, or other, adverse events.)

It's not helping matters that FDA now says it won't convene its advisory committee to discuss the data ahead of approving Pfizer's vaccine. (Last August, to address vaccine hesitancy, the agency had "committed to use an advisory committee composed of independent experts to ensure deliberations about authorization or licensure are transparent for the public.")

Prior to the preprint, my view, along with a group of around 30 clinicians, scientists, and patient advocates, was that there were simply too many open questions about all Covid-19 vaccines to support approving any this year. The preprint has, unfortunately, addressed

152 *Unblinding* is the moment of a clinical test in which data on who received the medicine and who the placebo are revealed (either to patients or to researchers).

> very few of those open questions, and has raised some new ones.
>
> I reiterate our call: "slow down and get the science right—there is no legitimate reason to hurry to grant a license to a coronavirus vaccine."
>
> FDA should be demanding that the companies complete the two year follow-up, as originally planned (even without a placebo group, much can still be learned about safety). They should demand adequate, controlled studies using patient outcomes in the now substantial population of people who have recovered from Covid. And regulators should bolster public trust by helping ensure that everyone can access the underlying data."[153]

This very strong reaction against the FDA's decision centers above all on the further exception that it has created in the vaccine approval processes. The first exception was the one that led to emergency approval. The second is not to wait for the expected time to evaluate the data on efficacy and risks before final approval. Let me also note that this way of proceeding has been characterized by a serious lack of transparency capable of generating distrust and hesitation towards the anti-Covid vaccines and towards the decisions of the competent agency.

8.1.1. Technical and Ethical Aspects

Now, on the technical aspects of this reaction to the double decision of the FDA – that is, to not make use, contrary to what was planned, of the independent scientific advisory body, and to

153 See P. Doshi, "Does the FDA think these data justify the first full approval of a covid-19 vaccine?," *BMJ*, August 23, 2021, URL: https://blogs.bmj.com/bmj/2021/08/23/does-the-fda-think-these-data-justify-the-first-full-approval-of-a-covid-19-vaccine/?fbclid=IwAR37TctCimlAauC912I-EUZVAMdudgaP0VKmGKmmu876JaB0xoMEMCfsxxA. The emphasis is mine.

give definitive approval to one of the vaccines available on the market by cutting the time planned for data verification – the experts in the fields involved could discuss at length and, of course, everyone could share or criticize every single point of this debate. On the other hand, from an ethical point of view and from the standpoint of moral reasoning (of all, both experts, professionals, and ordinary people), things are very different.

In fact, the debate that emerges from journals such as the BMJ does not present an alleged "world of science," on the one hand, and an alleged "world of the ignorant," on the other. This is a debate within science that sees recognized experts on both sides—some even within those same committees that are responsible for decisions and/or evaluations on vaccines. In other words, it is the same scientists who are experts in the relevant field who express doubts about anti-Covid vaccines and who criticize the lack of transparency and the politicization of the decisions of the government drug agencies. And it is the American government agency, the FDA itself, that recognized the presence of these problems when, precisely to stem the effect on the population, it had ensured the use of a committee of *independent* experts to evaluate and make better decisions (with calm awareness of the situation) regarding vaccine approval issues.

The logic of this last point is also somewhat odd. I think of all those easy critics who immediately lashed out at the BMJ reaction and in favor of the FDA, but without understanding that by doing so, they also criticized the FDA. In other words, it was initially the FDA itself that felt the need to consult independent scientists before making the most important decisions. This means that the FDA is sensitive to the issue and aware of the possibility that its decisions are not, or are accused of not being, transparent or independent, and therefore ultimately dictated not by science but by non-scientific reasons (political, economic, etc.). There is no escape from logic. If the BMJ is criticized on this point, at the same time, the FDA is also criticized. The FDA, at least from an ethical and deontological point of view, should provide an explanation for its change of course.

Doubt beat the virus to the punch. If with the virus, in fact, there is still the doubt that it may become endemic (although many scientists now take this for granted), with the doubt this doubt is no longer there. Doubt is now endemic to Covid vaccines. It could not have become so if the authorities had acted with full transparency and respect for the intelligence of citizens (from all over the world, not just from individual states), but it is now virtually impossible to restore a reasonable condition of trust, which unfortunately will irreparably damage the future relationship of ordinary people with drug authorities and any future vaccines.

8.2. Striking Resignations

But let's go back for a moment to the extra-scientific reasons that may have forced the FDA to grant full approval to the Pfizer vaccine by shortening the time of studies on the data and avoiding the independent scientific committee. The main reason, BMJ tells us, is that the US government intended to initiate mandates and booster doses in September. President Biden had in fact stated that he would make vaccines mandatory by September 20, 2021. Obviously, we cannot be certain that this is really the reason that led to the FDA decision of August 23. However, we can evaluate other clues.

Here some might immediately accuse me of conspiracy theory. Let me say, therefore, that I do not like conspiracy theory, but even less do I like the ignorant or dishonest people who accuse those who try to reflect on available clues of being conspiracy theorists. Reflection on clues is an essential, and often predominant, part of the method of any science. Even some theories of quantum physics rely on clues about the behavior of alleged subatomic waves or particles. Reasoning based on clues is so scientific that it is part of both the civil and criminal process of any modern state, and often leads *per se* to sentences when the clues are serious, precise, and concordant (as we say in legal jargon). There are just verdicts based not on direct evidence but on clues, if these are such as to allow a reasonably or prudent-based certain judgment on what happened. Anyone who is unable to understand this and uses conspiratorial slogans to block circumstantial reasoning is stupid, ignorant, fanatical, or in bad faith. The objections of people who immediately cry conspiracy are useless, pointless, and, for those who want to do science, must be decidedly and completely ignored.

I say it differently. From a logical-scientific or epistemological point of view, some conclusions based on clues are more certain than all the risk-benefit assessments of the FDA and the EMA based on the consideration of future unknowns of the effects of vaccines.

So, let's go back to our clues. A few days after the FDA's decision on Pfizer, two of the top FDA executives committed to Covid vaccines announced their resignations from the FDA. These are Marion Gruber, Ph.D., director of the FDA's Office of Vaccines Research and Review, and Philip Krause, Ph.D., deputy director of the same office. Of course, there are no official statements on the reasons for the resignations. Newspapers around the world, however, have had no doubts (a simple basic search on the internet about this is enough). The resignations were motivated by the pressure the Biden regime put on the agency to immediately proceed with booster doses of vaccines as early as September 20—the unacceptable last piece of a mosaic of undue pressure exerted by political forces on medical agencies.

MSNBC, for example, which is one of the world's leading news agencies, after recalling Gruber's research seniority and global prestige (who previously also worked on Ebola and Zika vaccines), and after recalling Biden's announcement on booster doses as of Sept. 20, points out that these are the agency's non-political resignations, and links them to two other famous (and shocking in pandemic-time) resignations from the CDC: those of Nancy Messonnier, Ph.D., director of the National Center for Immunization and Respiratory Diseases at the Centers for Disease Control and Prevention—the first to have warned about the seriousness and risks of Covid—and Anne Schuchat, Principal Deputy Director of the Centers for Disease Control and Prevention.

> "The planned departure of Gruber and Krause has been acknowledged inside and outside the agency as a loss for the globe, and there's a good amount of speculation that the White House jumping in front of the FDA was the final straw. That story is certainly plausible — but it is more likely that their decisions to leave reflect a growing tension between career officials who have been pushed to the brink and felt at times irrelevant or unsupported [...] Unexpected departures of credible nonpolitical staff have exacerbated tensions within crucial government agencies; the departures of Nancy Messonnier and Anne Schuchat at the Centers for Disease Control and Prevention came shortly after leadership changes prompted by Dr. Rochelle Walensky, Biden's CDC director. Such departures are not unusual when they occur over months or years in the normal pitter-patter of government. But when four scientists and physicians at two of the most important United States agencies leave during the middle of a pandemic with no ready transition plan or heirs apparent, there is clearly a need to look to the agencies' leadership. In this case, the FDA lacks the necessary leadership in the Office of the Commissioner, and the public will pay a price for it."[154]

154 See K. Patel, "Why these Covid vaccine scientists resigned from the FDA," in *MSNBC*, September 1, 2021, URL: https://www.msnbc.com/opinion/why-these-covid-vaccine-scientist-resigned-fda-n1278207.

8.3. The Criticism in *The Lancet* and the Rejection of the Booster Dose

The story, however, does not end there, but continues at an even faster pace in specialized journals and subsequent FDA decisions.

What exactly happened? It happened that, on September 13, 2021, the two FDA resigning scientists, Marion Gruber and Philip Krause (who, of course, will continue to serve in the agency, the first, it seems, until the end of October and the second, with duties also replacing the first, until the end of November or until the changing of the guard), together with sixteen other scientists signed an article in *The Lancet*, one of the oldest and most prestigious peer-reviewed medical journals in the world, in which they criticize the idea that we must proceed with booster doses for everyone.[155] It is a direct attack on Biden's announcement made without the support of science and anticipating or forcing ongoing assessments by agencies.

> "Although the idea of further reducing the number of COVID-19 cases by enhancing immunity in vaccinated people is appealing, <u>any decision</u> to do so <u>should be evidence-based</u> and consider the benefits and risks for individuals and society [...] Careful and public scrutiny of the <u>evolving data</u> will be needed to assure that <u>decisions</u> about boosting are <u>informed by reliable science more than by politics</u>."[156]

155 P. R. Krause, T. R. Fleming, R. Peto, I. M. Longini, J. P. Figueroa, J. A. C. Sterne, A. Cravioto, H. Rees, J. P. T. Higgins, I. Boutron, H. Pan, M. F. Gruber, N. Arora, F. Kazi, R. Gaspar, S. Swaminathan, M. J. Ryan, A.-M. Henao-Restrepo, "Considerations in boosting COVID-19 vaccine immune responses," *The Lancet*, September 13, 2021, URL, https://www.thelancet.com/journals/lancet/article/PIIS0140-6736(21)02046-8/fulltext.

156 Ibid. The emphasis is mine.

The article goes on to clarify that a booster may currently be discussed for individuals who have not been sufficiently protected by the first doses, but even in these cases it could happen that those same individuals would not receive any benefit from a further dose. Rather, in the face of this uncertain benefit, the risks of the vaccine both in and of itself and with respect to the loss of confidence in vaccines that could result, in general, from the occurrence of adverse events should be considered:

> "Although the benefits of primary COVID-19 vaccination clearly outweigh the risks, there could be risks if boosters are widely introduced too soon, or too frequently, especially with vaccines that can have immune-mediated side-effects (such as myocarditis, which is more common after the second dose of some mRNA vaccines, or Guillain-Barre syndrome, which has been associated with adenovirus-vectored COVID-19 vaccines). If unnecessary boosting causes significant adverse reactions, there could be implications for vaccine acceptance that go beyond COVID-19 vaccines. Thus, widespread boosting should be undertaken only if there is clear evidence that it is appropriate."[157]

Here there is a hint of cynicism and utilitarianism that is sadly frequent in the authorities (both political and medical) who deal with Covid vaccines in an institutional way. In fact, it seems that the possible occurrence of "significant adverse reactions" has for the authors of the article only one negative consequence, that of being able to damage the population's general faith in vaccines. The true damage of significant adverse reactions, that is, the death and serious illness of real people, does not seem worthy of an explicit mention. I am not saying, of course, that the authors of the article are monsters, but when you put things in writing, the primary concerns and priorities of the writer clearly

157 Ibid. The emphasis is mine.

emerge. In this case, these concerns and priorities do not include those poor people who die or become seriously ill from vaccines. In any case, even with this type of primary ethical priority (or poverty) focused on the abstract good of vaccines above people, the article recalls at various points the concerns about benefit risk assessments in the face of still uncertain scientific data:

> "[...] a very short-term protective effect would not necessarily imply worthwhile long-term benefit [...] If boosters (whether expressing original or variant antigens) are ultimately to be used, there will be a need to identify specific circumstances in which the direct and indirect benefits of doing so are, on balance, clearly beneficial. Additional research could help to define such circumstances. Furthermore, given the robust booster responses reported for some vaccines, adequate booster responses might be achievable at lower doses, potentially with reduced safety concerns. Given the data gaps, any wide deployment of boosters should be accompanied by a plan to gather reliable data about how well they are working and how safe they are."[158]

To be clear, and with all due respect to fanatics, none of the authors of this article is an anti-vaxxer. Indeed, the article expresses a clear faith in vaccines and a confidence in the efficacy of the first round of same, as well as in the fact that the benefits of their initial use outweighed the risks. I am not referring to this article in *The Lancet* either against or in favor of vaccines, or to support a continuity or technical contradiction between this article and the views of the BMJ on the hasty and procedural and ethical anomaly of the FDA decision of August 23, 2021.

I am only highlighting the continuity of a series of close events related to the FDA that demonstrate, on the one hand, a legitimate and varied debate among scientists regarding vaccines

158 Ibid. The emphasis is mine.

and, on the other, the consequences of an illegitimate politicization of processes that should respect the timeframes of science and not those of elections, political consensus, or panic attacks by some rulers and opinion leaders.

Indeed, from my point of view, the article in *The Lancet* is characterized by a final position of an ethical nature that should please the pro vaxxers, first of all. In fact, it says that, given the uncertainties about a possible booster for already vaccinated individuals (who could in the future benefit better, hypothetically, from more diluted doses or doses calibrated only on the variants), it would be much more appropriate and desirable to use the scarce doses currently available for other individuals in the world who have not yet had the opportunity to be vaccinated. This is a generally shared position which, of course, must be combined with the other circumstances surrounding the regular administration of vaccines: especially, that of giving priority to the most exposed individuals with the correct information and medical history.

In any case, the story we are telling does not end there (and it will probably not end until the end of the pandemic and beyond), because the article in *The Lancet* was strategically published a few days (on September 13, 2021) before a meeting of the FDA external advisory committee scheduled for September 17, 2021 (which would also be attended by Marion Gruber for the FDA): that is, a meeting of that same committee of independent scientists who had not been called in August, thus sparking the reaction we have seen from the *BMJ*. The agenda for September 17 was precisely the boosters announced by Biden and criticized in *The Lancet*.

This meeting must have been a blow to Biden, who can partly control the FDA but not the independent outside experts. It was not possible to avoid it, however, given the many and authoritative public reactions to the choice of August 23. In fact, the words with which Peter Marks, Director of the FDA's Center for Biologics Research and Evaluation, announced the next meeting of the Advisory Committee seem to be borrowed from the criticisms of the BMJ:

> "The administration recently announced a plan to prepare for additional COVID-19 vaccine doses, or 'boosters,' this fall, and a key part of that plan is FDA completing an independent evaluation and determination of the safety and effectiveness of these additional vaccine doses.
>
> The process for authorizing or approving the use of a booster dose of a COVID-19 vaccine involves each vaccine manufacturer submitting data pertaining to safety and effectiveness to the agency to support this use. The FDA is evaluating data submitted by Pfizer-BioNTech in a supplemental Biologics License Application for its COVID-19 vaccine and will discuss it with the agency's advisory committee to inform our decision-making. Should the data received from other manufacturers raise unique questions that would benefit from the committee's input, the agency intends to consider additional public discussions.
>
> A transparent, thorough and objective review of the data by the FDA is critical so that the medical community and the public continue to have confidence in the safety and effectiveness of COVID-19 vaccines. The FDA will review the supplemental application as expeditiously as possible, while still doing so in a thorough and science-based manner."[159]

The accusations of lack of transparency, of politicization, and of engendering mistrust must have had their effect.

159 See "FDA In Brief: FDA to Hold Advisory Committee Meeting to Discuss Pfizer-BioNTech's Application for COVID-19 Booster," September 1, 2021, URL: https://www.fda.gov/news-events/press-announcements/fda-brief-fda-hold-advisory-committee-meeting-discuss-pfizer-biontechs-application-covid-19-booster.

And the resignations of Marion Gruber and Philip Krause (still in service) probably made them no longer ignorable. Many observers envisioned a difficult decision by the Advisory Committee, certainly not by a large majority. It was not so. The Committee decided with virtual unanimity, redeeming science from politics. Voting took place on two questions.

After a discussion of about 7 hours, during which the Committee analyzed Pfizer's request, accompanied by all the clinical tests of the case,[160] the first vote was reached on the following first question:

> "Voting question n. 1: Do the safety and effectiveness data from clinical trial C4591001 support approval of COMIRNATY booster dose administered at least 6 months after completion of the primary series for use in individuals 16 years of age and older?"[161]

To this question, the Committee voted no, with only two votes against out of 18 participants. This decision was expected by several experts, who had highlighted how Pfizer's request was based on extremely limited and exploratory data, with

---

160 See "FDA Briefing Document. Application for licensure of a booster dose for COMIRNATY (COVID-19 Vaccine, mRNA)," URL: https://www.fda.gov/media/152176/download. "Pfizer: Evaluation of a Booster Dose (Third Dose). Vaccines and Related Biological Products Advisory Committee Meeting. Meeting date: 17 September 2021," URL: https://www.fda.gov/media/152161/download.

161 To be prudent with respect to Covid, the meeting of the Committee took place remotely but was made available to the public on various platforms. See FDA, URL: https://www.fda.gov/advisory-committees/advisory-committee-calendar/vaccines-and-related-biological-products-advisory-committee-september-17-2021-meeting-announcement. This is the meeting link on YouTube: https://www.youtube.com/watch?v=WFph7-6t34M.

clinical tests on just over 300 people (only 11 for the over 65 age group).[162] The second question was the following:

> "Question n. 2: Based on the totality of available scientific evidence, including safety and efficacy data from clinical trial C4591001, the known and potential benefits outweigh the known and potential risks of a booster dose of Pfizer-BioNTech COVID-19 vaccine administered at least 6 months after completion of the primary series: in individuals aged 65 and over, and in individuals at high risk of severe COVID-19?"

To this second question, the Committee voted yes unanimously. A further discussion was then generated on the possibility that the third dose could also be recommended to those who are in conditions of particular exposure to Covid or who carry out jobs that are particularly high risk, as is the case with healthcare professionals. Peter Marks then reminded the Committee that their vote is not binding on the FDA and that, precisely for this reason, despite not being part of the question and the vote, it would have been interesting to hear the views of the members on this further aspect of the matter. With regard to referring in general to those who are in conditions of particular risk from exposure, there was the objection that this could apply to anyone and would therefore be a circumstance too subject to interpretation. With regard to particularly high-risk jobs, the personal opinion of the members was favorable.

This last personal opinion expressed by the members of the Committee leaves me quite perplexed. The negative vote on the first question was based above all on the fact that there is not

---

162 See, e.g., Ph.D. G. Poland's opinion, Mayo Clinic Vaccine Research Group Director (https://www.mayo.edu/research/faculty/poland-gregory-a-m-d/bio-00078220), expressed during the meeting of the Committee in the following interview: https://www.foxbusiness.com/healthcare/pfizer-covid-vaccine-kids.

enough data to say both that a third dose offers greater protection against the virus and that it cannot have negative effects greater than its supposed positive effects. The decision on the second question is therefore based on a sort of bet justified by the risk/benefit ratio linked to age (which makes long-term risks less relevant) and medical diseases, which makes people particularly vulnerable to Covid. The Committee also complained about the lack of data broken down by age group.

Personal opinions on the categories that carry out high-risk jobs seem, however, linked more to extra-scientific feelings and attitudes than to the data analyzed for the first question. This creates uncertainty as to what data is actually available to experts and the technical reasoning used to express opinions. Why, for example, should a twenty-year-old, even if engaged in jobs with a higher risk of contagion (in whatever way they are defined), who is in perfect health, who uses all prudent means to avoid contagion, and who would not run particular risks even from a possible contagion, submit to the uncertainty of the third dose given what was said by the experts in voting on the first question? It is interesting that the discussion on this point took place without further in-depth analysis, in a couple of minutes and at the end of a meeting of more than eight hours. From an epistemological point of view, I would say that the discourse fell in an instant from the scientific level to that of a chat over coffee not comparable even to poorly argued guesswork.

In general, it is interesting that the discussion of the Committee, in addition to highlighting the general lack of data available to support the decision on the first question, also called for a clearer differentiation or indication of data by age group, as well as the inconvenience of making decisions on ages thus defined in a context of variable data and situations. It was particularly amusing when one of the members said that, being 63, he would have preferred a question based on 60 rather than 65, adding essentially that this type of question leaves no room for prudent-based assessments of concrete cases of individuals at risk.

The discussions of the members of such a committee are very far from the fictitious certainties and the inability to problematize and reflect that sadly characterizes political proclamations and television studios. It is also interesting that the Committee's scholars, even when expressing conflicting opinions, did not insult or harshly criticize each other. This marks the difference between experts and TV studio screamers.

In any case, predictably, the FDA's formal decision on the issues discussed by the Scientific Committee was in line with expert opinion. In fact, on September 22, 2021, the FDA communicated its formal decision to allow a "single booster dose" of the Pfizer vaccine, "to be administered at least six months after the completion of the primary series," to the following categories of subjects:

> "individuals 65 years of age and older;
> individuals 18 through 64 years of age at high risk of severe COVID-19; and
> individuals 18 through 64 years of age whose frequent institutional or occupational exposure to SARS-CoV-2 puts them at high risk of serious complications of COVID-19 including severe COVID-19."[163]

163 See FDA, "FDA Authorizes Booster Dose of Pfizer-BioNTech COVID-19 Vaccine for Certain Populations," September 22, 2021, URL: https://www.fda.gov/news-events/press-announcements/fda-authorizes-booster-dose-pfizer-biontech-covid-19-vaccine-certain-populations: "Today, the U.S. Food and Drug Administration amended the emergency use authorization (EUA) for the Pfizer-BioNTech COVID-19 Vaccine to allow for use of a single booster dose, to be administered at least six months after completion of the primary series in: individuals 65 years of age and older; individuals 18 through 64 years of age at high risk of severe COVID-19; and individuals 18 through 64 years of age whose frequent institutional or occupational exposure to SARS-CoV-2 puts them at high risk of serious complications of COVID-19 including severe COVID-19."

It should be noted that this authorization was carried out as an addition to the emergency one (EUA) and not as an addition to the full authorization, confirming the scientific uncertainty of the same and the double track line for the Pfizer vaccine.

8.4. The Humiliation of the CDC Committee

During the meeting of the Scientific Committee of the FDA, Sara Oliver, a representative of the CDC (Centers for Disease Control and Prevention), was also connected in streaming with the members to give a presentation on the epidemiology of vaccines and took an active part in the discussion.[164]

---

164 It is worth remembering that, in her presentation, Oliver reported a table showing a strong difference between the hospitalizations of vaccinated and unvaccinated. The latter were far superior. This is very important for pharmaceutical companies as emergency authorizations are also based on the assumption that vaccines reduce hospitalizations. The same data reported by Oliver had been used by President Biden and the Director of the CDC, Rochelle Walensky, to publicly speak of Covid-19 as an "epidemic of the unvaccinated". However, the data in Oliver's table were based on a reference period ranging from 01/24/2021 to 07/17/2021, and it is obvious that in the first part of the year the number of unvaccinated was far greater to the vaccinated. Consider, for example, that in March the vaccinated with double dose increased from 7.8% to 16.6%, and that at the end of April they were still 30.9%. The number of double-dose vaccinates will reach 50% of the population only on 07/30/2021, i.e., after the reference period considered by Oliver. There was considerable public controversy over this misuse of statistical data. See, for example, the report on Fox News with an interview with virologist Byram Bridle, URL: https://video.foxnews.com/v/6266738894001#sp=show-clips. Prof. Bridle, after having publicly expressed his perplexities about vaccines, in particular about the fact that they could have negative repercussions on the heart, suffered strong media and work persecution, to the point that he denounced harassment even in the workplace. See, e.g., K. Arm-

(continued on the next page)

It is noteworthy that a few days after the meeting of the Committee and two days after the official decision of the FDA, that is, on September 24, 2021, the Advisory Committee of the CDC met to deliberate on the same matter. This committee,

a) voted unanimously to allow the booster for people over 65 or in retirement homes,
b) voted 13 to 2 to allow it for people aged 50 to 64 with medical conditions such as to raise the risk of a serious Covid-19 infection, and
c) voted nine to six to allow it for people between 18 and 49 with medical problems.

In other words, the advisory committee of the CDC had strong certainties about the third dose for the elderly, fewer certainties about the third dose for those at risk between 50 and 64, and much fewer for those, even with medical problems, under 50. The line of thinking is clear enough, but definitely at odds with Biden's political aspirations. On the same day, therefore, with a rare and striking move, the director of the CDC, Rochelle Walensky (nominated by the president) decided to disregard the opinion of the Committee to further enlarge the audience of candidates for the third dose.[165]

---

strong, "U of G prof says he is receiving workplace harassment after sharing vaccine concerns," *Guelphtoday*, June 19, 2021, URL: https://www.guelphtoday.com/local-news/u-of-g-prof-says-he-is-receiving-workplace-harassment-after-sharing-vaccine-concerns-3888634.

165 See, e.g., B. Lovelace, Jr., R. Towei, "The leader of CDC just made a rare call to allow Covid booster shots for more people," *CNBC*, September 23, 2021, URL: https://www.cnbc.com/2021/09/23/covid-booster-shots-cdc-panel-endorses-third-pfizer-doses-for-millions.html; H. Keene, "CDC's COVID booster shot reversal: Is the Biden administration following the science?," *Fox News*, September 24, 2021, URL: https://www.foxnews.com/politics/cdc-covid-booster-shot-reversal-biden-administration-following-science.

Still, Walensky's decision remained broadly in line (with minimal non-substantial differences) with that of the FDA, recommending booster doses

a) for individuals over 65,
b) for those over 18 in care facilities,
c) for those between 50 and 64 with particular medical conditions, and adding that such doses may also be received
d) by subjects between 18 and 49 with particular medical conditions, and
e) by those exposed to greater risk of contagion because of their job.[166]

Of course, the White House was shouting victory, after the humiliation that came from the FDA, in this surreal conflict and storyline between politics, science, and pharmaceutical companies.

8.5. The EMA's Decision on Third Doses and Booster Doses

As I said before, the history of decisions on vaccines almost always sees Europe following American choices by a few weeks, often extending their scope to more vaccines or more cases. Interestingly, the case of additional doses is also no exception.

Indeed, on October 4, 2021, less than two weeks after the FDA and CDC decisions, the EMA's Committee for Medicinal Products for Human Use (CHMP) decided to recommend

166 See CDC (Centers for Disease Control and Prevention), "Pfizer-BioNTech COVID-19 Vaccine Booster Shot," Updated Sept. 24, 2021, URL: https://www.cdc.gov/coronavirus/2019-ncov/vaccines/booster-shot.html.

both booster and extra doses with Pfizer's vaccine (Comirnaty) and with Spikevax Moderna.[167]

More specifically, the EMA stressed the importance of distinguishing "between the extra dose for people with weakened immune systems and booster doses for people with normal immune systems."[168] The extra dose (of Pfizer or Moderna) was just recommended by the EMA (at least 28 days after the second dose) for only people with weakened immune systems. Booster doses, on the other hand, were recommended (only with Pfizer and at least six months after the second dose) for all subjects over 18 years of age. I will have to return elsewhere to the specific characteristics of these recommendations and their subsequent developments.

8.6. The CDC Changes the Definition of "Vaccine"

I have to take a step back now to talk about a humorous debate that has arisen in connection with the fact that the US CDC recently changed the definition of vaccine. It's funny because it was like watching, during a football game in which a team gains a yard, the sprawled reaction of the opposing supporters standing up to unleash their best counter wave and their best slogans for their team in difficulty. Seeing science reduced to opposing supporters is so depressing that laughing at it is the only comforting solution. What exactly happened?

It happened that, between late August and early September of 2021, the CDC changed its definitions of what vaccination is. The case was brought to the attention of the media above all by a September 8 tweet from Thomas Massie (a Repub-

167 See "Comirnaty and Spikevax: EMA recommendations on extra doses and boosters," News October 4, 2021, URL: https://www.ema.europa.eu/en/news/comirnaty-spikevax-ema-recommendations-extra-doses-boosters.

168 Ibid.

lican politician from Kentucky) which in a short time exceeded 20,000 likes and 12,000 retweets.[169] Massie's tweet was polemic (bolstered by a reference to Orwell that only culture lovers, of all sides, can appreciate), but it was also very simple as it only reported the evolution of the CDC vaccination definitions before 2015, between 2015 and 2021, and from September 2021. Here they are:

> "Vaccination (pre-2015): Injection of a killed or a weakened infectious organism in order to **prevent** the disease.
>
> Vaccination (2015-2021): The act of introducing a vaccine into the body to produce **immunity** to a specific disease.
>
> Vaccination (Sept 2021): The act of introducing a vaccine into the body to produce **protection** from a specific disease."[170]

The first definition still mirrors the commonsense notion of a vaccine, similar to the traditional concept that if you take small doses of a poison, you can become immune to it. It also reflects the commonsense notion that the vaccine, unlike other drugs, is administered to the healthy to prevent disease, and not to the sick. That notion actually seemed antiquated. Today there are apparently also vaccines—such as those with purified immunogens or antigens or with anatoxins—that do not inject the virus as such (dead or weakened); and there are post-exposure prophylaxis vaccines—such as rabies, or measles and chickenpox vaccines—that are also given to those who are already sick to elicit a faster immune reaction before the virus reaches the nervous system.

---

169 See T. Massie, "Check out @CDCgov's evolving definition of "vaccination"," URL: https://twitter.com/RepThomasMassie/status/1435606845926871041/photo/1.

170 Ibid.

The necessary evolution of vaccine science, however, was, for the CDC, inversely proportional to the will to define it. Clearly, the post-2015 definitions of "vaccination" no longer have a defining character. In fact, when vaccination is defined as the administration of a vaccine, a mere tautology is applied which refers to the definition of vaccine. To be clear: if we define "coloring" in terms of "using colors," we only express the difference between the noun and the verbal form of something, but nothing is said of what it is. The pre-2015 definition was antiquated but definitory; the subsequent ones only tell us that both the noun and the verb exist for a certain thing.

Still, all the definitions express the purpose of vaccination: to prevent, immunize, protect. But let's go back for a moment to the controversies between supporters. There are so many fans out there that I just need to pick one at random from the mainstream media that immediately felt the need to respond to Massie. *The Washington Post* is the winner.

From the columns of this newspaper, the morning after Massie's tweet, Aaron Blake takes up what happened by explaining that, behind Massie's post, there is the idea that the CDC has diluted its definition because the anti-Covid vaccines have proved less effective than expected. Blake acknowledges that "it's interesting that the CDC changed the Web page," but "as for the conclusions being drawn about its significance?" he has nothing to say. His only concern is to explain that no vaccine protects 100% and that immunity, in medicine, is only synonymous with protection. To do this, he even goes to the trouble of checking the language dictionaries and other pages of the CDC from which it appears that immunity simply means protection.

This display of dictionaries from the *Washington Post* is woefully useless. The author of the article does not even realize the difference between protecting (or making immune) from a virus and a disease. So, let's leave the supporters alone and go back to the CDC. Let's see if, nominalisms aside, there is really something interesting here to understand.

8.6.1. Vaccine, Vaccination, Immunity, and Immunization

First of all, let's broaden the discussion a little instead of limiting it to the evolution of the concept of vaccination. In fact, on the pertinent page of the CDC we are offered four definitions:

> "Definition of Terms:
>
> **Immunity:** Protection from an infectious disease. If you are immune to a disease, you can be exposed to it without becoming infected.
>
> **Vaccine:** A preparation that is used to stimulate the body's immune response against diseases. Vaccines are usually administered through needle injections, but some can be administered by mouth or sprayed into the nose.
>
> **Vaccination:** The act of introducing a vaccine into the body to produce protection from a specific disease.
>
> **Immunization:** A process by which a person becomes protected against a disease through vaccination. This term is often used interchangeably with vaccination or inoculation."[171]

In this page of the CDC, the first thing evident to a third party observer is the theoretical interest in linking the concepts of immunity and vaccine and, consequently, those of immunization and vaccination as verbs expressing the actions that have as their object, respectively, immunity and the vaccine. From the point of view of systematic interpretation, this is an indubitable architectural starting point.

The other indubitable fact concerns the definition of immunity, which corresponds well to the commonsense concept of total protection from a certain infection: "If you are immune to a disease, you can be exposed to it without becoming infect-

171 See CDC, "Immunization: The Basics," URL: https://www.cdc.gov/vaccines/vac-gen/imz-basics.htm.

ed." Probably, at the *Washington Post*, in their haste, they didn't even look at the most relevant page of the CDC. They went straight from the tweet to Google searches.

The third indubitable fact is the logical link between immunization and vaccine. Immunization is a process that occurs through vaccination, to the point that the two terms are often used interchangeably. Immunity (whatever it is) is achieved through the vaccine (whatever it is). Blake was right about one thing: that immunization and protection are synonymous here. He was wrong, however, that they do not indicate 100% protection.

The fourth indubitable fact is that the CDC has renounced a content-based or substantial definition of the vaccine in favor of a mere functional definition. Previously, the vaccine was defined on the basis of what was injected (the dead or weakened infected organism). Now, it is defined only as a "preparation" which fulfills a certain purpose. As I said, this definition appears more correct with respect to the evolution of vaccine science. I advise the CDC to also update their internal dictionary, still the child of past science and which would not allow the inclusion of both anti-Covid and new generation vaccines among the vaccines.

> "**Vaccine**: A suspension of live (usually attenuated) or inactivated microorganisms (e.g. bacteria or viruses) or fractions thereof administered to induce immunity and prevent infectious diseases and their sequelae. Some vaccines contain highly defined antigens (e.g., the polysaccharide of *Haemophilus influenzae* type b or the surface antigen of hepatitis B); others have antigens that are complex or incompletely defined (e.g. *Bordetella pertussis* antigens or live attenuated viruses)."[172]

172 See CDC, "Glossary," URL: https://www.cdc.gov/vaccines/terms/glossary.html.

Of course, if this definition of the CDC Glossary were not an error due to the failure to update, we would have to insert it into our systematic interpretation of the CDC and conclude that "preparation," in the definition of vaccine on the previous page, means "suspension of live (usually attenuated) or inactivated microorganisms (e.g. bacteria or viruses) or fractions." We should also conclude that the purpose of the vaccine can also be expressed in this way, to "induce immunity and prevent infectious diseases and their sequelae." In this case, both the changes noted by Massie, that of 2015 and that of 2021, would ultimately be irrelevant stylistic updates, and many new generation vaccines (including anti-Covid ones) would continue to fall outside the CDC definition of a vaccine.

The fifth indubitable fact that emerges is that the CDC creates a significant logical confusion between the definitions of vaccine and vaccination. The vaccine is of course a tool and cannot be defined independently of the purpose for which it is produced and used. The CDC definition of a vaccine therefore includes both the act of using it ("a preparation that is used") and the purpose of its use ("to stimulate the body's immune response against diseases"). But the act of using the vaccine is called vaccination and the purpose of using the vaccine must therefore correspond to the purpose of vaccination.

The CDC, however, has decided to define vaccination using different terms, which is confusing. On the one hand, it says that vaccination is the act of using the vaccine, and this is tautological, useless, but correct. On the other hand, however, it expresses the purpose of vaccination in different words than those used to express the purpose of the vaccine. Vaccination, says the CDC, is done to "to produce protection from a specific disease." A third party observer must therefore assume that these two things, "[stimulating] the body's immune response against diseases" and "[producing] protection from a specific disease," coincide. This is a logical, venial sin but still a sin. The first element indicates in fact the modality in which the vaccine operates, the second the aim. Both have definitional value.

Apart from the logical confusion in exposing the concepts, there are apparently no particular problems here. I suggest that the CDC, for the next update, define the vaccine as “a preparation that is intended to generate protection from a specific disease by stimulating the body’s immune response against it.” Or, using the purpose expressed in the Glossary: “a preparation that is intended to induce immunity and prevent infectious diseases and their consequences, and which works by stimulating the body’s immune response against them.” This second seems to me to be more informative and adequate. The term “is intended to” is more correct than “is used” because it expresses the very purpose for which the vaccine is produced. A hammer can be used as a paperweight but is not built for it. Use, *per se*, does not define the thing. The vaccine, like the hammer, is produced for a specific purpose that determines its use (at least the main or ordinary one). Therefore, a good definition of the vaccine must contain the purpose for which it is manufactured/used and how it works (by stimulating the immune system).

8.6.2. A Deceptive but Logically Irrelevant Change

Let's pretend we know absolutely nothing about the controversy between fans and the recent change of definition made by the CDC. Let’s see exactly what we can logically deduce from what we read in the four definitions of the CDC.

1) That the CDC does not know how to define vaccine and vaccination adequately and without creating confusion,
2) That the CDC has given up (at least on that web page) on a content-based definition of the vaccine.
3) That the purpose of the vaccine and of vaccination is to generate protection from a specific disease by stimulating the body’s immune response against it,

4) That immunity offers such protection that if you are exposed to that disease, you will not be infected,
5) That immunity is achieved through vaccination to the point that the two terms are treated as synonyms,
6) That the current anti-Covid vaccines are not definable as vaccines based on the systematic logical interpretation of the current definitions of the CDC.

According to the logic of the definitions offered by the CDC, therefore, we can deduce that the recent change has no real meaning. Here, too, Blake, in spite of himself, was right. So why change it and why in this period? To answer these questions, I must abandon the logical sense that emerges from that page of the CDC and work with clues. Let me emphasize that for the moment this discourse has a circumstantial nature and a weak truth value. It's interesting, though, because it seems to me more likely that the CDC truly wanted to change something in the definition (no time is wasted on prose and poetry while a pandemic emergency is in progress), but that it has done so in a way so clumsy that it did not have (at least until the next change) any effect whatsoever.

It seems to me that there are sufficient indications that the CDC, more than the FDA, wants to favor Biden's policy in the direction of increasing additional doses and mandatory vaccination. However, it is unrealistic to impose a mandate with vaccines under emergency authorizations, and it is obvious that Pfizer's authorization has lowered the scientific bar on vaccines both in terms of safety and efficacy.

That the CDC has tried to dilute the concept of immunity through that of protection, in this context, seems to me the most plausible rational assumption, and it is interesting that pro-vaccine supporters like Blake understood it this way, essentially and precisely defending this lowering of the bar.

It is obvious that immunity in medical vaccine science cannot be understood as a mathematical absolute, but that it tends towards a qualified concept of absoluteness is equally obvious. From this point of view, there is no doubt that Pfizer's approval and the idea of mandatory vaccination are favored by a dilution of the ideal of vaccine immunity. The CDC probably wanted to make a first timid and strategic move in the direction of this lowering of standards, but it did it in a clumsy and incomplete way. We will see if it continues in this direction.

The difference between a virus (Sars-Cov-2) and a disease (Covid) must also be considered. The two things do not coincide and there has been much too much confusion with respect to them. The traditional concept of a vaccine protects against the virus, not the disease. Those who are vaccinated do not get infected, that is, they do not contract the disease. The efficacy of the new anti-Covid vaccines, however, has never been seriously tested and/or guaranteed with respect to contagion. These pseudo vaccines have not been placed on the market to protect against contagion, or to confer immunity. Their alleged efficacy, the only one of which something can (in theory and roughly) be guaranteed, concerns the symptoms of Covid disease, in the sense that those who are vaccinated should run less risk from the disease than those who are not vaccinated. From this point of view, it is obvious (politically, not scientifically) that the CDC felt the need to dilute, on the one hand, the definition of vaccine and the boundary between immunity and protection and, on the other, those between viruses and disease.

8.6.3. The Deception Comes to Light

In the previous section I worked with clues, which reflects the historical drafting of this book, the chapters of which were all drafted before October 2021. Now, however, there is no longer a need to use too much imagination because, thanks to a FOIA, unambiguous documents emerged concerning the real reasons for the CDC's clumsy efforts with definitions of vaccine and vaccination.

It is Thomas Massie himself who, in a tweet from November 5, 2021, confirms that, following a FOIA (appeal for access to documents under the Freedom of Information Act), proof has been obtained that the CDC has changed the definition of vaccine without any scientific basis, only to include the new anti-Covid vaccines.[173]

See, in particular, an internal CDC email of August 25, 2021, addressed to a certain Valerie Morelli, which reads:

> "Hi Valerie, I know you are busy so I really appreciate your help. The definition of vaccine we have posted is problematic and people are using it to claim that COVID-19 vaccine is not a vaccine based on our own definition. Does the updated version look okay to you?
> Currently posted:
> **Vaccine**: A product that stimulates a person's immune system to produce immunity to a specific disease, protecting the person from that disease. Vaccines are usually administered through needle injections, but can also be administered by mouth or sprayed into the nose.
> Update to
> **Vaccine**: A preparation that is used to stimulate the body's immune response against diseases. Vaccines are usually administered through needle injections, but can also be administered by mouth or sprayed into the nose."[174]

---

173 See T. Massie, tweet November 05, 2021, URL: https://twitter.com/RepThomasMassie/status/14566789115601100 80.

174 See *Il Paragone*, "Il CDC Usa cambia la definizione scientifica di "vaccino" per farci rientrare quello anti-Covid," November 30, 2021, URL: https://www.ilparagone.it/attualita/cdc-cambia-definizione-vaccino/?fbclid=IwAR0UG4epirpT1X5dcNV_v3gXldgZTSzCqq_YKea0ZamlkwWV_obnOAhJijY.

On September 1, 2021, Alycia E. Downs, of the CDC, writes a new email to Valerie asking for confirmation of the change in the definition of "vaccination."

> "Does this definition need to be updated as well?
>
> **Vaccination**: The act of introducing a vaccine into the body to produce immunity to a specific disease.
>
> To something like:
>
> **Vaccination**: The act of introducing a vaccine into the body to produce protection from a specific disease."[175]

To this new message, Valerie replies on the same day as follows:

"If this is for the general public I am good with the change."[176]

The intent to dilute the concept of immunity—and of vaccine in general—to protect anti-Covid vaccines from attacks by *vile deniers* is now clear; as it is clear that there is no science and study behind this change, only demagogic political strategy. Valerie's latest response, from this point of view, is both enlightening and disturbing. In fact, it implies the existence of a double truth or a double level of scientific study, as if to say that if that change is for the ignorant and irrelevant people of the general public, then the change is fine. If, on the other hand, it should have a scientific basis, then it would be appropriate to work on it seriously. This, at least, seems to be the most reasonable interpretation of that type of answer.

Note in this exchange the clarity with which the intent to empty the defining concepts for the general public emerges (in order to better protect themselves from any attack) specifically with the elimination of the reference to the disease. In short, these CDC geniuses (geniuses in the sense that they do not belong to the vulgar general public) have thought of something like this: "And if the anti-Covid vaccines did not have a real efficacy,

175 Ibid.

176 Ibid.

not only against the virus, but also against Covid? Let's do it this way then, let's just define that the vaccine is a preparation (that is, anything) that is introduced into the body to stimulate a response of the immune system against diseases in general." Brilliant! Who will ever be able to prove that the Covid vaccine is not a vaccine if it is sufficient, for this purpose, to produce any effect in the immune system that generically protects against any disease or symptom of it? Anything we put into the body will cause some immune system reaction or stimulus. How sad, Valerie! Alycia, what a shame!

8.6.4. The General Risks of These Changes in Definitions

I would like to dwell—aside from the pro-vaxxer and anti-vaxxer supporters, aside from the Blake-like articles and from the defining gossip of the CDC (because this is what those changes in definition amount to)—on two possible risks of this tendency to lower the bar on Covid vaccines and to dilute the concepts of vaccine and immunization to the advantage of protection. To clarify: I don't care right now if the CDC made that change as part of a broader strategy, whether political or of another type. I don't care right now about the problem of Covid vaccines as such. I believe, instead, that the debate that has been created is useful for reflecting in general on these problems, and reflecting is always an important thing.

8.6.4.1. Obligatory Medicines for the Healthy

Vaccines have a fundamental characteristic that differentiates them from other drugs: with some exceptions, they are given to the healthy and not to the sick. Selling medicines to the healthy is of course the dream of any pharmaceutical company, as Henry Gadsden, CEO of Merck, famously told Fortune magazine years ago.[177] But that's not the point (or it's not the only point). The point is that vaccines, due to their immunizing efficacy, are often made mandatory for very serious diseases. Other vaccines, such as meningococcus, always worry any parent a lot, but it is often decided to obtain them, even if/when they are not mandatory (and waiting for a while with bated breath), precisely because they offer a very high level of protection.

Now, precisely because it is a medicine for healthy people, the vaccine should be adequately and prudently limited to cases in which there is a state of necessity prudently defined by law (both in synchronic and diachronic terms) and a reasonable (very high) efficacy that justifies both the risks associated with the use of the vaccine and the restriction of the personal freedom of citizens in matters affecting their health and that of their loved ones.

Let's do a thought experiment now. Let's pretend we're a cynical pharmaceutical company executive whose sole goal is to increase profit, whatever the cost. I am not saying that we get to the point of carrying out illegal experiments on Nigerian children,[178] but yes, that we intend to stop at nothing. What strategy

---

177 On this, of course, the well-known book by Ray Moynihan and Alan Cassels should be read, *Selling Sickness: How the World's Biggest Pharmaceutical Companies Are Turning Us All into Patients* (Nation Books: New York, NY 2005). See also M. Petersen, *Our Daily Meds: How the Pharmaceutical Companies Transformed Themselves into Slick Marketing Machines and Hooked the Nation on Prescription Drugs* (Picador: New York, 2009); C. Lane, *Shyness: How Normal Behavior Became a Sickness* (Yale University Press: New Haven, 2007).

178 *BBC*, "Pfizer: Nigeria drug trial victims get compensation," August 11, 2021, URL: https://www.bbc.com/news/world-africa-14493277; *The New York Times*, "*Nigerians Receive First Payments for Children Who Died in 1996 Meningitis Drug Trial*," August 11, 2021, URL: https://www.nytimes.com/2011/08/12/world/africa/12nigeria.html; Forbes, "Pfizer's Nigerian Nightmare," November 20, 2008, URL: https://www.forbes.com/forbes/2008/1208/066.html?sh=5a11d7623

(continued on the next page)

should such a character adopt with respect to vaccines to achieve the goal of selling more to the healthy? Simple, it should do the following two things:

a) Dilute the concept of vaccine so that it can generically include any product that can provide some help against a disease, and
b) Eliminate the idea that the vaccine must provide immunity (albeit within the reasonable limits that this concept can assume in medical science).

Such a strategy could certainly favor the current anti-Covid vaccines because, of course, there are no stable certainties on their efficacy over both the short and long term. But it would be absolutely perfect for a hypothetical future in which there will be many other products which, while not guaranteeing immunity in any way, could be presented as vaccines and perhaps even made mandatory by law.

To avoid a future of this type, however imaginative or realistic it may really be, it is obvious that we must maintain, both epistemologically and ethically, a high standard of the concept of vaccine—a standard that is best guaranteed by the use of the term and concept of "immunity." When my wife and I had our little boy receive the meningococcal vaccine, we knew perfectly well that it did not mathematically guarantee 100% protection, but the concept of immunity as such was not questioned. It is not mathematics that questions this medical health concept; it is the hypothesis of changing it now and the reasons for doing so.

a71; The Guardian, "Pfizer pays out to Nigerian families of meningitis drug trial victims," August 12, 2011, URL: https://www.theguardian.com/world/2011/aug/11/pfizer-nigeria-meningitis-drug-compensation.

8.6.4.2. Everything Becomes a Potential Vaccine

Let's focus now on the first element of that strategy, that of diluting the concept of vaccine so that it can generically include any product that can provide some help against a disease.

We have seen that this trend is already present in the recent definition change made by the CDC, even if somewhat mitigated by the presence of the old definition in the Glossary. We have also seen that some definitional change could be required by the evolution of vaccine science—but with regard to the virus not to the disease. Depriving the concept of vaccine of any content trait does not seem correct, but referring to the vaccine not as protection against a virus, but as protection against the symptoms of any disease is a move that undermines any sensible concept of vaccine. A serious definitional effort must be made here because by separating the concept of vaccine from those of immunity and viruses, everything becomes or can become a vaccine.

If the vaccine is any "preparation" meant to "stimulate the immune response" or "produce protection from a specific disease" or "induce immunity and prevent infectious diseases and their sequelae" (I use the three goals/ends of the CDC that we have just seen), what distinguishes the vaccine from any preparation meant to prevent, or even – assuming the removal of the term "preparation" in the future - from any prevention criterion? If vitamin D, for example, truly had some efficacy against Covid, why shouldn't it be considered a vaccine? And if it were effective to rest, to sleep well, or to reduce symptoms, why couldn't a sleeping pill, a day home from work or the gym, or an aspirin be considered a vaccine?

Whoever thinks I am exaggerating does not understand logic, does not know history, and has no imagination. Let me say it again, therefore: the end alone does not define the instrument. The purpose of the vaccine cannot be only to combat the symptoms of any disease, and a definition based on the purpose alone will necessarily end up including anything that can somehow serve that purpose. If I say that "X is for sitting," I have not communicated anything about what X is, and whatever helps one to sit, from a chair to a freight elevator or to a team of nurses that lifts the patient and takes him to a chair, will fall into X. If you want to define the chair, it is not enough to state its use.

Defining the vaccine well with respect to both its purpose and its content is important both for the law and for pharmaceutical companies. And it is also important for those who in the future will have to choose whether to use a vaccine or simple, more or less effective, prevention tools.

8.6.4.3. The Merriam-Webster Definition Change

In a recent round table organized by Wisconsin Senator Ron Johnson, Peter Doshi highlighted that even the well-known American dictionary Merriam-Webster, in 2021, changed its definition of vaccine twice, in January and October: the definition had not been touched since 2006.[179] Merriam-Webster's changes are in line with the CDC's phony science. The first change, in January, eliminates the content, passing from "a preparation of [...] organisms" to simply "a preparation," and adds below (in case there is any doubt about the reasons for the change) two points ("a" and "b") on mRNA preparations and on the spike

179 On Senator Johnson's YouTube channel, which was initially censored by the super scientist YouTube for this very roundtable, there is a video of it in which, however, Doshi's discussion is not reported in full. For some reason, space was given only to the second part of the intervention dedicated to the lack of transparency of vaccine data: see, "Vaccine Mandates Expert Panel Highlights held by Sen. Ron Johnson," November 2, 2021, URL: https://www.youtube.com/watch?v=lkVN3KwDfvI. Doshi's full lecture, in which he also addresses the change in the definition of vaccine, can be heard, for example, here, https://brandnewtube.com/watch/peter-doshi-u-s-senator-ron-johnson-holds-panel-in-dc-on-covid-19-vaccine-mandates-and-injuries_LWTWpHPVdy2Ye6U.html. I thank Peter Doshi for privately sending me the slides of the presentation.

protein. Leaving aside the specifications of points "a" and "b," this is the change of definition we witness in January 2021:

> **January 18, 2006**:
> "A preparation of killed microorganisms, living attenuated organisms, or living fully virulent organisms that is administered to produce or artificially increase immunity to a particular disease."
>
> **January 26, 2021**:
> "A preparation that is administered (as by injection) to stimulate the body's immune response against a specific infectious disease."

The logic of the change is clear and twofold: the content is eliminated and the reference to immunity is eliminated. Maybe Merriam-Webster asked Valerie and Alycia for advice. Who knows? The second change, that of October, further modifies the definition and adds a second alternative to the first. We now have definition 1 and definition 2.

> **October 23, 2021**:
>
> 1. "A preparation that is administered (as by injection) to stimulate the body's immune response against a specific infectious agent or disease."
> 2. "A preparation or immunotherapy that is used to stimulate the body's immune response against noninfectious substances, agents, or diseases."

Here it should first be noted that definition no. 1 is changed by adding "infectious agent" to "infectious disease." In this way the concept of vaccine is emancipated from the concept of disease. Any infectious agent (such as a bacterium or a protozoan), even if it does not constitute an infectious disease, can be something to be vaccinated against. Of course, if we assume that an infectious agent could cause infections and diseases, this specification could still make logical and medical sense. But let's look at definition no. 2.

Here we have first of all the addition (to "preparation") of immunotherapy, which is an innovative cancer treatment based in general on the idea of treating the cancer cell as if it were a virus or an infection to be eradicated by the immune system. Immunotherapy involves injecting drugs (such as Ipilimumab, Pembrolizumab, Nivolumab and Atezolizumab) into the body, sometimes directly into cancer cells.

In reality, in medical oncology literature, immunotherapy does not necessarily coincide, from a conceptual point of view, with the innovative idea of a cancer vaccine. This is how, for example, the Cancer Treatment Centers of America explains it:

"How does immunotherapy spark the immune system to help fight cancer?

> Immunotherapies use different methods to attack tumor cells. Immunotherapy types fall into three general categories:
>
> - Checkpoint inhibitors, where cancer cell signals that trick the immune system into thinking they're healthy cells are disrupted, exposing them to attack by the immune system.
> - Cytokines, where protein molecules called cytokines—those that help regulate and direct the immune system—are synthesized in a laboratory and then injected into the body in much larger doses than are produced naturally.
> - Cancer vaccines, which may reduce the risk of cancer by attacking viruses that cause cancer, or may treat cancer by stimulating the immune system to attack cancer cells in a specific part of the body.

> Immunotherapy may be used alone or in combination with other cancer treatments, such as surgery, chemotherapy, radiation therapy and targeted therapy."[180]

The idea of a cancer vaccine is therefore in a relationship of part to whole with respect to immunotherapies and has a dual aspect. On the one hand, it is a normal vaccine that acts against a virus that could cause cancer: that is, it is not a true vaccine against cancer, but a vaccine that, given the virus against which it operates, also constitutes a prevention against cancer. The only vaccine of this type currently in circulation is the one against the papillomavirus, which is a virus that "can cause health problems like genital warts and cancer."[181] With respect to cancer, this type of vaccine is called prophylactic or preventive but, of course, it would not require immunotherapies to be included in the notion of vaccine. On the other hand, there are so-called therapeutic vaccines: those that, as I said above, conceptually treat the tumor as if it were a virus and require treatments with weekly dosages that can be repeated for months or even a year.

Definition n. 2 of Merriam-Webster is so broad with respect to immunotherapies as to not only include those that, in the fight against cancer, would not be called vaccines today, but also to consider vaccines therapies with weekly, monthly or annual dosages.

Let us now move on to the second part of the definition which, on the one hand, eliminates the mode of injection, suggesting that the vaccine could also be given in pills or surgically introduced into the body, and, on the other hand, modifies the

---

180 See *Cancer Treatment Centers of America*, "Immunoterapy," updated on September 21, 2021, URL: https://www.cancercenter.com/treatment-options/precision-medicine/immunotherapy.

181 See CDC, "Genital HPV Infection – Fact Sheet," Last reviewed: January 3, 2022, URL: https://www.cdc.gov/std/hpv/stdfact-hpv.htm.

end, which is no longer just fighting an infectious disease or an agent that causes it, but also fighting "noninfectious substances." According to this definition, therefore, a vaccine is also any product introduced into the body in any way with any therapeutic regularity and for the purpose of fighting anything, even a non-infectious substance.

If I were a psychologist, I would try to positively interpret Merriam-Webster's intentions by hypothesizing that the addition of "noninfectious substances" is directed to a product aimed at destroying cancer cells. However, I am not a psychologist but a logician and an ethicist, and I see infinite problems with this dilution of the notion of a vaccine which deprives it *in fact and in law* of any specificity that would identify it as something different from the others. A definition that does not distinguish what is defined from other things, however, is no longer a definition. In the case of medical and health issues, it is a time bomb. Frankly, the ease with which entities in 2021 like the CDC and Merriam-Webster, caught by some sort of frenetic ideology or Covid-vaccine promotion syndrome, have started this process of progressive destruction of the concept of vaccine, is incomprehensible to me.

In his speech at Johnson's round table, Doshi wonders how we would have reacted to the idea of mandatory vaccination if these new products—which do not prevent infection or transmission of the virus—were not called vaccines but simply drugs. If the only thing they do, allegedly (and as long as people get them with constant and unpredictable cyclicality), is to alleviate certain consequences of a disease, why not consider them like any other drug and include them with others that help us when we are sick? Doshi's question brings us back to the political and ethical-legal importance of the "vaccine" brand, which should maintain very precise teleological and content/efficacy-related features if it is to continue to make sense in the legal and health system.

The efficacy of anti-Covid vaccines, as I have already pointed out, is perhaps the most striking aspect of the weak science behind them. The variable and contradictory news and announcements that we have seen in the last year on the efficacy of these products are more suitable for a variety program than for a scientific discussion. The weak science of efficacy has given way to another weak science, that of additional booster doses. And on these too, an irregular syncopated dance between decreasing efficacy and multiplying of doses has begun. These days, we are starting to address with concern the fact that the succession of doses could damage the immune system, perhaps irreparably. We would thus have a vaccine (we hope not) that not only fails to guarantee immunity from a disease, not only fails to protect against infections and the transmission of the virus, not only fails to provide guarantees of efficacy over time, but even damages the entire immune structure of the human being.

Was it really necessary to panic and call it a vaccine? Was it really necessary to start an unscientific and conceptually unsustainable process to crumble the definition of "vaccine" to the point of making it meaningless? Was it really necessary to engender such distrust in medical science? And to say that it would have been enough, with a pinch of humility and common sense, to tell the population exactly what we had and to try with maturity to use it to the fullest, recognizing its limits.

This is not the time when the miracle occurred of producing Covid vaccines in record time. This is the period when medical science has achieved an unrivaled record of contradictory, false, and imprudent information on a weekly, if not daily basis. A period in which something that is scientific in one state or to one expert is not scientific in another state or to another expert. A period in which international politics promulgated the strength of weak science, putting it at the basis of the worst campaign of persecution and violation of the rights of the individual ever seen, at least in such a widespread and surreptitiously invasive way. This is a period that unfortunately will be very difficult to leave behind.

8.7. "Emergency Authorizations": Epistemological Remarks

I now want to summarize the most important epistemological aspects relating to the circumstance of the marketing of anti-Covid vaccines through emergency authorizations, of which, in this and in the previous chapters, I have outlined the legal, ethical, scientific, and epistemological aspects.

We should remember that this circumstance is very much intertwined with the previous one on risks, which I discussed in chapter 4, as well as with the specific conditions of the authorizations which I will have to postpone to a future volume. What makes emergency authorization a specific circumstance for moral conscience is the fact that it possesses its own autonomy based on a specific legal nature. The mere fact that the law proceeds with the emergency authorization of one or more products has an impact on the agent's ethical reasoning, regardless of the significance of other circumstances.

Let me also recall, as already done in the last chapter, that this type of summary is functional to the ethical assessments of the specific circumstance under discussion, and that there is not always a direct correspondence between individual epistemological findings and individual ethical consequences.

1. **Legal nature of emergency authorizations**
   The emergency authorizations of the FDA and the EMA have a legal nature, even if they concern areas that belong to medical and scientific disciplines. The decisions of the FDA and the EMA on such authorizations involve legal, ethical, and political, and not just scientific, processes and evaluations. It is highly misleading to look at the FDA and the EMA as if they were just authoritative voices, like many others, in the world of science.

2. **Experimental vaccines**
   The very nature of emergency vaccine authorizations implies incomplete data to be completed in the future. This, in a technical sense, means that at the time of the emergency authorization, knowledge about the vaccines is not yet solidified from the point of view of experimental science, and that, to become so, experiments will have to continue after the authorizations. In the general explanations on the meaning and requirements of the emergency authorization, the FDA appears less clear than the EMA on incomplete or absent data. However, the FDA is much clearer than the EMA on the same issue in the detailed information on individual vaccines.
3. **Authorization requirements**
   Emergency authorizations imply specific conditions or criteria without which authorization cannot be given or loses meaning. These criteria must be evaluated one by one both in a synchronic and diachronic sense. It is necessary to verify with which scientific principles and arguments their existence and certainty have been assessed, as well as the criteria that determine their termination.
4. **Conflict of interest**
   The studies and data underlying the anti-Covid vaccines are produced by the same pharmaceutical companies interested in the approval or authorization of the product. This does not make them fully reliable. The provisional reliability criterion to be used with pharmaceutical companies also depends on the trust that can be placed in them with respect to their history and their known policies and behavioral practices.
5. **Limits of the scientific world**
   It must also be considered that the scientific world, even in the post-emergency authorization phase, cannot enter into full synergy with the vaccine studies of pharmaceutical companies because many data on vaccines are protected by

industrial secrecy. Pharmaceutical companies don't share all information. This fact maintains an imbalance between the studies and data of companies in conflict of interest, which are more complete but less reliable and certain, and the studies and data of independent science, which are more reliable but less complete and therefore of equally doubtful certainty. This year we will see the impact on the scientific community of the first FOIA regarding the authorization documents of one of the vaccines (Pfizer) which should be fully available by 2022.

6. **Special reliability of the truths of the law**
   The legal profiles related to vaccines—from emergency authorizations to pharmaceutical company contracts and to special regulations such as the Italian criminal shield and American immunity—possess a greater degree of certainty than the statements, even by experts, made freely in other contexts that do not imply direct assumption of responsibility. In the case of Covid vaccines, the law pinpoints the state of uncertainty and risk recognized even by the pharmaceutical manufacturers.
7. **Pfizer's final approval**
   The decision relating to this approval is surrounded by the more than reasonable doubt that it was risky and unfounded from a scientific point of view and dictated only by political reasons in support of the Biden administration. It is reasonable to assume that the FDA Advisory Committee was not convened to avoid public discussion and to avoid being bound by a negative opinion from independent experts. It is noteworthy that, in this case, unlike the others, the EMA did not follow the example of the FDA. We are therefore facing a case of divergence of views on the same vaccine and on the basis of the same data by two of the most important world government agencies. The scientific truth-value of the FDA approval is almost nil, both because it is not supported by similar decisions by other international

agencies and because of the strong immediate criticism from important sectors of the independent scientific world. It should also be kept in mind that, in the face of a critique published in a major journal, there are thousands of similar expert opinions that have not been published. The division within the world of science, in this case, is quite evident.

8. **Change of vaccine definition**
   The clumsy attempt to change the definition of a vaccine to include the new Covid vaccines is not based on science but on politics and business. Technically, the current change in definition of the CDC, despite the intentions of the authors, does not allow the current anti-Covid products to be defined as vaccines. Ongoing attempts to change the definition of a vaccine risk completely nullifying its logical and conceptual meaning. For the purpose of an adequate definition, both the content of the product and its purpose, as well as what distinguishes it from other drugs and medical therapies, must be carefully considered.

8.8. "Emergency Authorizations": Ethical Consequences

Let me now shift the focus to the ethical consequences of this circumstance. Naturally, to summarize these consequences I will also use the specific epistemological findings just reviewed.

1. **Vaccines available not by science but by law**
   Those who approach the possible choice of Covid vaccines must consider that they are currently available, not due to a definitive judgment from science, but due to an emergency decision of a political nature and on the basis of emergency legislation.
2. **Legal and political uncertainty**
   Those who approach the possible choice of the vaccine must know that the political authorities do not have strong certainties in this regard, and that this is what emerges une-

quivocally from the official documents and from the emergency regulations. Any certainties displayed by someone in the media are a scam or, in very few cases, a mistake made in good faith by ignorant people.

3. **Right to information**
   Citizens must be informed that the anti-Covid vaccines have been approved, not according to the times and rules of ordinary protocols, but according to emergency criteria that imply missing data and require constant updating, testing, and monitoring studies.
4. **Serious doubt**
   Emergency authorizations, due to the epistemological limits that characterize them, in themselves entail a very serious state of doubt for the moral subject: a state of doubt that must be carefully evaluated.
5. **Experimental vaccines**
   Anyone who approaches the possible choice of vaccines should know that they are experimental with respect to the medium and long term both in terms of efficacy and, and above all, in terms of potential negative effects. They are also partly experimental in the short term, which is why all forecasts on the timing and efficacy of vaccine protection have not worked and are constantly changing. Experimental science does not fail in comparison with facts, because it is the comparison with facts that previously founded it as an experimental science. If vaccine predictions have failed even in the medium term, this is proof that they had not been tested, or that they had been using limited and provisional science.
6. **Full approval of Pfizer**
   Anyone approaching the possible choice of vaccines should know that there is currently a single vaccine that has been given full approval by the American FDA alone, and that this authorization is not valid in other parts of the world and has been strongly criticized by a respectable and author-

itative part of the world of science. The most correct ethical attitude is to doubt the validity and seriousness of this authorization.

7. **Like an emergency authorization**
   The final approval of Pfizer, given the negligible value of scientific certainty that surrounds it, and since it is not corroborated by similar decisions of other international agencies, does not give any guarantee to moral conscience. From an ethical point of view, even for those who live in the United States of America, it is better to consider the Pfizer vaccine like any other Covid vaccine in emergency use without giving weight to its final approval by the FDA.
8. **Intertwining of politics and science**
   Those who approach the possible choice of vaccines should know that there are strong pressures and influences exerted by politics on the agencies responsible for authorizing drugs and vaccines, and that, precisely in relation to that one vaccine that has been fully approved, a considerable tension between science and politics was immediately generated. With respect to this problem, the task of those who must make the ethical choice is not the (impossible) one of expressing an opinion on who is right (the FDA, the Advisory Committee, the Biden Presidency, the BMJ, etc.). The problem is simply to understand the merit and scope of the relevant discussions in the world of science and politics. The moral conscience will have to take note of these things and express itself in some way about them.
9. **Authorization requirements**
   Before deciding to take one of the so-called Covid vaccines, the moral conscience must assess whether, at the specific time and territory, the conditions for the emergency use of the vaccine still exist.
10. **Conflict of interest**
   Those who approach the choice of one of the vaccines must also consider that the initial studies, still predominant, and

many of the follow-up studies are produced in conflict of interest by the manufacturers themselves, and therefore have a lower level of reliability than the studies produced by independent science. The moral subject must question the reliability of the relevant manufacturer.

11. **Non-decisive circumstance**
    The circumstance *per se* of the authorization for the emergency use of a vaccine cannot of course be decisive for the moral conscience, both because the norm itself provides for the freedom of choice of the vaccine and because this circumstance says nothing, as such, about the specific limits and administration criteria with respect to specific pathologies and people.
12. **Vaccine mandate**
    The nature of the current authorizations of the so-called Covid vaccines, coupled with the fact that their testing is still ongoing and with the fact that all the presumptively scientific information on their efficacy and safety has proved fallacious and unreliable (changing from month to month and week by week), makes any vaccine mandate unsuitable. The very idea of providing for such compulsion is contrary to the fundamental principles of medical ethics and the experimentation of drugs and therapies on human beings. The surreptitious attempt of many legislations around the world to create indirect vaccine mandates by threatening the unvaccinated population or preventing them from accessing public services and the exercise of fundamental rights and freedoms is highly immoral and reveals a dangerous utilitarian and totalitarian political drift. The social hatred and violence that is spreading in many countries should be an ethical priority for the moral consciences of both ordinary citizens and especially those with political and governmental responsibilities.
13. **Definition of vaccine**

The surreptitious attempt to change the definition of a vaccine to protect current Covid vaccines is highly immoral. The very use of the term vaccine for these products has been immoral and is at the origin of almost all the problems of informed consent and social political tension that have surrounded the debate on them since they were placed on the market and mandated. A correct ethical attitude should lead the competent agencies and sector experts to question themselves on what should be an adequate definition of a vaccine that respects both its technical and political ethical requirements. In fact, the term "vaccine" should enjoy particular public reliability, and be reserved for products to which, due to their characteristics of efficacy and reliability, special legal implications can be connected.

Conclusion

Although the writing of this book preceded that of *The Death of the Phronimos: Faith and Truth About Anti Covid Vaccines*, this conclusion follows its publication by several weeks. I waited until the last moment to write it, until the last drafts were corrected and sent to the publisher for printing. It seems like a century has passed since that first publication, but it has only been a few months. The times of emergency make the succession of facts and information move so quickly that even new and recent things soon appear old.

The *Confessions* of Saint Augustine come to mind. In particular, the eleventh book, which contains perhaps the most beautiful text ever written on the concept of time. The past no longer exists, therefore it does not have a duration because what is not cannot last. The duration of the past belongs to the soul. When it seems to us that a century has passed since a certain event, it is because other events so important and oppressive that they have already clouded our memory of it have followed. The same book, the same movie, the same music are too short if we like them (they finish too soon) and too long if we don't like them (they never end). Two months seem like a century when we have run too much on an unpleasant track, when the whole world has run too far on that track and can't wait for it to end. When the soul does not have time to consider something sufficiently because so many other matters emerge—important, urgent, and crucial—that thing fades in the memory and appears increasingly distant. The soul's attention to new events, the impossibility of remaining in the memory of the past, makes the past more and more past.

In these days of fast-paced hectic events, I see above all three new and curious phenomena in the landscape of the pandemic. One I'll call the worried wise guys' phenomenon. The other two are bizarre because they are inversely proportional to each other. I start with these.

The book *The Death of the Phronimos* closed with an escalation, especially in the persecutory and despotic tenor of the provisions of the political authorities of many countries. This exaggerated escalation—beyond my expectations, I must say—is certainly one of the characterizing events of this time. In Canada they want to institute a general tax on the unvaccinated—as an exemplary punishment, evidently, which satisfies the sense of revenge of those who have completed their *act of love*. Fauci would like swabs for all healthy people in the United States. In Australia, they no longer know what else to do and focus their anger on a tennis player—a person who had also donated a lot of money at the beginning of the epidemic to help the first seriously infected, but who does not intend to get vaccinated and is therefore intrinsically incapable of acts of love. Macron *bursts with love* from every pore and says he wants to "*emmerder*" the unvaccinated. As president he is not that great, but in this (in putting all of us into a pile of excrement), it must be said that he was very good.

In Italy, they invented the *super green pass* (super vaccine passport), which for example prevents people like me from having coffee at the bar (even standing up) and imprisons them/us on an island (Sicily) because leaving it would involve taking a plane or a ferry, which, like all means of public transportation, are forbidden to those belonging to the *sanitary race* of the unvaccinated. I will have a conference in Rome in the coming months. In order to attend, I'll have to rent a dinghy from Libya. On the other hand, as a reward, vaccinated people infected with the virus no longer need to quarantine and can go around freely to infect the population. I could go on—the examples are countless. But this is not a cabaret book, to laugh together at the political performances in the various states, nor a psychiatry book, full of therapies for collective psychosis or that of individual leaders, nor a book of religion or sociology, to analyze the collective belief in the vaccine god.

The peculiar thing about this psychotic escalation of governmental control is that it is moving in the opposite direction of the pandemic. The Omicron variant is at the root of the neurotic panic of the latest escalation, but it is a variant in itself that is not very problematic, and everyone is beginning to understand it. Some experts even consider it a natural vaccine, because it is very contagious but not very dangerous, with the advantage that those who get sick could become immune to the virus in general without running particular risks (including the unpredictable ones that result from the pseudo vaccines). A worse variant of Delta would have been dramatic, but Omicron seems more like a positive sign of the end of the pandemic. In a sense, it might be better to hope that everyone will get infected with it, and that authorities will distribute information on what to do to react to the disease and how to overcome it better, rather than the ineffective precautions and pseudo vaccines. The idea of rushing to produce a new specific vaccine for Omicron, which may arrive when this variant is now a thing of the past, is like a therapeutic obstinacy of the drunken politics of the last year.

The road of vaccines and booster doses begins to appear to everyone as the worst path to take. The schizophrenia of information on the efficacy of vaccines that has been provided for a year now is increasingly emerging, with varying efficacy from week to week—a sign of official science that is weak and adrift. Herd immunity showed the incompetence of those who tried to predict it and to convince the population that it would be reached within a few months with 60% of the vaccinated, or rather 70%, or perhaps 80% or 85%, in fact 90%, or that's it, let's do it 100% and then we won't have to talk about it anymore. The fact is that it is precisely the most vaccinated countries (the richest ones) that suffer most from the pandemic and the new waves of infections. Political reaction centered only on the vaccine god to the detriment of any other preventative measure, starting with the effective treatments of primary care doctors and early therapies, has shown its failure in the most ignominious way and now, like a wounded animal, it growls and thrashes. Will these also be new signs of the billions of *acts of love* performed in this upside-down world? For those who keep themselves informed, it is evident that in the mainstream media there is fear that the house of cards is about to collapse, and a different and more complex or open vision of reality is starting to break through. Lies, they say, have short legs, and the ones about these pseudo vaccines have stretched their little legs forward as far as they can.

Here enter the worried wise guys, which are the journalists and those alleged experts who in 2021 were public preachers of the faith in the vaccine god, but who now perceive a potential near future in which they will be proven wrong and be humiliated—a future in which the absurdities, the weakness, and the contradictions of what was presented by them as "science" will appear in all its inconsistency and, why not, bad faith. These crafty and worried hypocrites are changing some of their views these days by trying to appear more moderate and *scientific*. They want to distance themselves from pro-vaxxer fanaticism. They warn that the end of the pandemic is near, that the failure of the vaccine policy is near, and they want to try to come out of it as winners, moderate, cautious. No one, however, even among those who were forced to get vaccinated and among those who are now disappointed or who have suffered adverse effects, seems willing to easily forget.

Perhaps the reason for this inversely proportional movement of the phenomena I have just described is that those who have the power of *official* science and communication cleverly think of saving themselves by gradually starting to appear more moderate and honest, while those with the power of government cleverly think of saving themselves by hoping that the end of the pandemic coincides with the period of greatest Jacobin rigor of their action and precedes the moment when the vaccines will prove definitively fallacious. The hope is to be able to say soon, perhaps thanks to Omicron and before the umpteenth joke about the failed efficacy of vaccines: "You see? Thanks to our extreme measures we have defeated the pandemic." The different approach also reflects the different liability risks. After all, TV experts and journalists have to fear looking foolish in the face of public opinion. Politicians in government, on the other hand, could suffer much more serious consequences related to repeated lies, manipulation of information, persecutory or undemocratic acts, and serious negligence.

We could almost laugh at it if it weren't for the fact that the Jacobin fury of the vaccine god has reached the children, who clearly derive no benefit from these experimental products but rather many unpredictable damages. I pray that despite the biggest deceptive media campaign ever seen in the modern world, many parents manage to keep a cautious approach and so save their children from this cynical and immoral experimentation.

In recent days, an Italian bishop has absolutely forbidden those in his diocese to visit the elderly and the sick without a reinforced vaccine passport (green pass). This is the bleakest example that comes to my mind of a church in disarray that kneels before other gods. These are the most dramatic fruits of the idea of the vaccine as an act of love.

On the other hand, I have also recently seen splendid examples of solidarity and of commitment to truth and love both inside and outside the Church. I have seen heroic priests who look people in the eye and dispense the supernatural fruits of their ministry regardless of pandemic panic and vaccine wars. I have seen scientists and experts working hard to help everyone recover a fair and honest relationship with real facts and problems. I have seen lawyers and jurists coordinating their efforts to react against this huge global violation of the fundamental rights of the person and of the democratic order. I have seen independent journalists trying to insert different and authoritative voices into the public debate. I have seen doctors loudly and repeatedly renew the Hippocratic Oath, despite a policy committed to reducing medicine to the material administration of pseudo salvific drugs. I have seen fellow philosophers, theologians, and ethicists from all over the world stand up and get to work to recover depth in the relationship between the world and the spirit, and to defend the truth.

Veritas vincit!
Veritas liberabit vos!
Omnia vincit amor!

Fulvio Di Blasi
Palermo, January 28, 2022
Feast of St. Thomas Aquinas

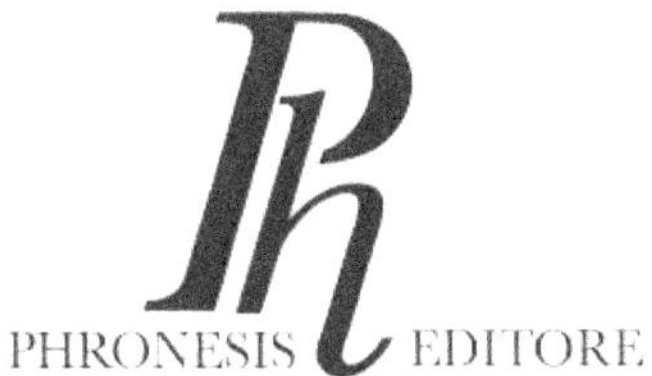
PHRONESIS EDITORE

www.ingramcontent.com/pod-product-compliance
Lightning Source LLC
LaVergne TN
LVHW020053210726
843507LV00016B/2109

* 9 7 8 8 8 9 7 3 2 8 3 7 7 *